Working with Fathers

Mary Ryan

Research Development Consultant

Radcliffe Medical Press

Radcliffe Medical Press Ltd
18 Marcham Road, Abingdon, Oxon OX14 1AA

British Library Cataloguing in Publication Data

A catalogue record for this book is available from the British Library.

ISBN 1 85775 487 5

Typeset by Acorn Bookwork, Salisbury, Wilts.
Printed and bound by TJ International Ltd, Padstow, Cornwall

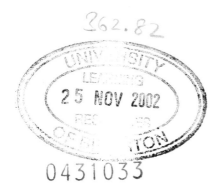

Contents

Chapter 1

Introduction

There is currently much interest in fathers, particularly among policy makers who are trying to keep pace with the changing roles of men and women in the home. Are things changing too far and too fast? What policies are needed to accommodate change or alternatively to bolster more traditional roles? In order to answer these questions, it is necessary to establish just what impact on their children's development fathers have when they are in the home and when they are elsewhere.

Academic observers point out that the interest in the role of fathers is not new and that there has been a steady stream of papers, particularly looking at fathers' impact on child development, since the 1930s (Lewis and O'Brien, 1987; Lamb, 1997). In the introduction to the third edition of *The Role of the Father in Child Development*, Lamb comments that at the time of the publication of the first edition in the mid-1970s, social scientists, particularly developmental psychologists, doubted whether fathers had any significant role to play in the development of their children. Now there is widespread acceptance that they do have a significant impact and an increasing volume of studies are looking at more complex and specific aspects of their role. Research in the area of fathers' influence on child development indicates that where there is a high level of paternal involvement, by agreement between the parents, the children have increased cognitive competence, perform better socially and academically, and have less sex-stereotyped beliefs. These findings are unsurprising and are related to the fact that such children have two involved adults providing diversity of stimulation and, sometimes, different parenting styles. In such families there are also less likely to be gender-stereotyped roles. Importantly, the research indicates that it is the characteristics of the father as a **parent** rather than as a **man** which are most significant, thus the important dimensions of parental influence are those which have to do with parental rather than gender characteristics (Lamb, 1997).

Researchers and commentators also note that while much is written about fathers and their impact on child development and their role in the family, relatively little research has been done on their influence in families where children are showing signs of disturbance or on fathers who are violent to their partners and/or maltreat their children (Phares, 1996; Sternberg, 1997). Similarly, in the social work field, while there appears to have been a recognition for some time that fathers are important and that they are insufficiently engaged by practitioners, this interest in the role of fathers has to date had little impact on the way in which social workers and other childcare practitioners work with families referred to social services; the focus has remained firmly on mothers and their ability to care for or protect their children (Marsh, 1987; Ruxton, 1992; Burgess and Ruxton, 1996; O'Hagan and Dillenburger, 1995).

Child Protection: messages from research (Department of Health, 1995a) summarised findings from 20 studies commissioned in the light of the 1987 Cleveland Inquiry. Not all of the findings found their way into print in that form as there was a limit to what could be captured. Moreover, organising the findings so as to draw attention to general themes meant that important points of detail had to be overlooked – one of which was the area of work with fathers.

The aim here is to inform practitioners working with children in need and their families what these research studies have to say about fathers and the professional response to them. The researchers were not asked to look specifically at fathers or at ways of engaging or working with them but the studies did contain sufficient information on fathers to draw out some general themes and messages. The particular studies from which this information has been drawn are listed in the Appendix (*see* page 81).

The main research studies that inform this paper focused on families involved in the child protection process at some stage – ranging from families where there was a suspicion or allegation of abuse leading to an initial enquiry, through those cases where there was a child protection conference to those where the child's name was placed on the child protection register (*see* page 21 for a brief explanation of the child protection system). The studies did not look at families in contact with social services departments where protection issues had not been the reason for the referral or contact, in other words, children and families coming within the wider definition of 'in need' in the *Children Act 1989*. The information on fathers contained in the studies has thus been collected from families where there are higher levels of professional concerns about child protection and where one would expect to find high levels of need and complex problems. Information on the normative studies disseminated through *Child Protection: messages from research* (Nobes and Smith, 1997; 2000) has been included in the section on context which follows.

Other research, or overviews of research, from both the UK and the USA, have been drawn on to provide context and information about different ways of working with fathers. In addition, this book contains information about projects that entail working with fathers, in relation to specific issues or generally, to provide some examples for practice. Although some of these projects have been evaluated, they have not been specifically evaluated by the Department of Health.

Before looking in detail at the findings from the studies that concern fathers, this book sets the information in context by considering more general socio-demographic information on fathers and families and the relevant legal provisions. The first question to ask is what do we mean by the term 'father'? Here it is applied to men living in the home with children and having some sort of father-type relationship with them, also to men outside the home – non-resident fathers – who have a biological or legal relationship with children in the home, or who had a caring role in relation to the children when they lived there. The tortuous nature of this definition is an example of the complex family relationships with which practitioners have to deal.

Issues for future research

The exercise of collecting information from the research studies has highlighted certain important issues for further research, issues already familiar to those studying the impact of fathers and fathers' roles in relation to troubled children and needy families (Phares, 1997; Sternberg, 1997). They show the importance of future research:

- distinguishing between mothers and fathers in order to identify who was interviewed and whom the observation concerns
- distinguishing between fathers and stepfathers
- distinguishing between fathers and father figures
- distinguishing between the abusing and the non-abusing parent
- collecting information from fathers as well as from professionals, mothers and children
- collecting information on fathers from different minority ethnic groups
- assessing how fathers perceive services on offer to children and families
- assessing how far services identify and meet the needs of fathers.

Chapter 2

Context: Fatherhood in general

The socio-demographic picture

There is surprisingly little data on the socio-demography of fatherhood. The best sources are the Office of National Statistics (ONS, 1997) publication *Social Focus on Families* and the Family Policy Studies Centre's *Fathers and Fatherhood in Britain* (Burghes *et al.*, 1997). The latter publication pulls together research information on the economic role of fathers and their contribution to the emotional, psychological and social development of their children, and as such is an extremely useful source of information. It draws heavily on the British Household Panel Study (BHPS, 1992).

Men and fatherhood

There are some 28 million men in Britain of whom 22 million are potential or actual fathers. The BHPS found that three-fifths (61%) of the men in its sample of 4350 had fathered a child and around half of these had dependent children under the age of 18.

It is generally the case that families with children have the father of the children living at home with them. In 1995–96, 75% of families with children were headed by a couple and 93% of these couples were married. The majority of births reported by men in the BHPS occurred within marriage, although a higher proportion (nearly 17%) of recent births, between 1986 and 1991, were reported as occurring outside marriage. In 1998, 43.7% of the births registered in

England and Wales were outside marriage (ONS, 2000). More than four out of every five fathers (84%) live with all their children under the age of 18, 73% of these fathers are living in their first family situation, 5% are lone fathers and 6% are in a subsequent relationship. Only a minority had two or more families. Family type does vary depending on the age of the head of the family, social class, geographical location and ethnicity of the family (ONS, 1997).

These findings set the wide coverage of the rise in lone parenthood in the UK in context. In 1995–96, 22% of all families with children were headed by a lone parent and 20% of dependent children were living in such situations.

Lone fathers

While there has been an increase in lone parenthood, the proportion of lone fathers has remained fairly stable for the past 30 years. There are nine lone mothers for every lone father and, not surprisingly, the profile of each contrasts. Lone fathers tend to look after older children; nearly a fifth (17%) of their offspring are aged 16 and over with three-quarters aged ten years or more (by comparison, just 30% of children of lone mothers fall into the same age category). Just 6% of lone fathers' children are below school age compared with a third (36%) of lone mothers' children.

Lone fathers are usually older than lone mothers. Nine out of ten (compared with just four in ten of the mothers) are aged 35 years or more. It is unsurprising, therefore, to find that the circumstances of lone fathers are somewhat different from those of lone mothers. There are more widowed than single lone fathers (for lone mothers the ratio is one to seven). Nearly half of lone fathers are divorced and another third (29%) are separated from their partners. The situation of children living with lone fathers tends to change more quickly than those living with lone mothers; one in ten each year cease to be dependent (reflecting the older age of children living with lone fathers) and 6% leave home. Just under one in ten of lone fathers remarry or begin a cohabiting relationship each year (ONS, 1997).

Step-parents

There has been an increase in step-parenting over the past 30 years but, again, it is relatively uncommon for children to live in step-parent households. Some 7% of families with dependent children comprise a step-parent and a natural parent. The great majority of step-parents are male. Only one in ten of parents in step-parent households is the birth father of one of the children compared with nearly nine in ten (86%) who are the birth mother.

Non-resident fathers

With lone motherhood and step-fathers now being present in just over a quarter (28%) of households with dependent offspring, there are many more fathers than ever before living away from their children. However, the picture of absent, unsupporting fathers is less common than might be supposed. Nearly half (47%) of non-resident fathers surveyed by the Social Policy Research Unit at the University of York saw their children at least once a month with two-thirds (68%) of these in contact more regularly than this. Only 3% of non-resident fathers have lost touch with their children altogether, with another 18% seeing their offspring less than once a year (Bradshaw *et al.*, 1997). The National Child Development Study showed that seven in ten fathers who did not live with their children at that time nonetheless had contact with them (Clarke, 1997).

Fathers' economic role

Traditionally the role of fathers has been as breadwinner while mothers have cared for the home and family. This view is supported by legislation such as the *Child Support Act 1991*, focusing on fathers' responsibility to maintain their families financially. This traditional division of labour in the home has been much criticised by feminist theorists over recent decades and more recently policy makers have been concerning themselves with fathers' roles as carers of their children rather than simply focusing on breadwinning. In March 1992, the Council of Ministers of the European Communities published its *Recommendation on Child Care*. Article 6 of the Recommendation states:

> As regards responsibilities arising from the care and upbringing of children, it is recommended that Member States should promote and encourage, with due respect for freedom of the individual, increased participation by men, in order to achieve a more equal sharing of parental responsibilities between men and women and to enable women to have a more effective role in the labour market.

In 1994, the European Commission's White Paper on Social Policy highlighted the need 'to relieve the burden (of family responsibilities) on women and allow men to play a more fulfilling role in society'.

The Family Policy Studies Centre notes that according to the British Social Attitudes Survey of 1992, just over a half of British men (53%) and 42% of women agree that 'a husband's job is to earn money; a wife's job is to look after the home and family'. In other words, almost a half of British men do not support a traditional breadwinning model, although the evidence indicates that fathers are still the main breadwinners in the majority of families.

The Family Policy Studies Centre's work indicates that employment rates for resident fathers have been consistently high since the beginning of the 1980s. It is estimated that nearly nine in ten fathers are in employment and nine out of ten of these occupations are full time. However, unemployment among young men generally has risen in recent years and among young fathers is even higher, so that almost half of the fathers aged 20–24 in the 1992 BHPS were unemployed. Given that the breadwinning role of fathers remains important, these figures raise issues for policy makers in relation to the barriers faced by young fathers in carrying out their traditional roles, let alone when taking on new ones. It could also be argued that the possibility of them taking on new roles is greater when they do not have to face the barriers imposed by employers or their work environment.

Compared with those in two-parent families, lone fathers are less likely to be in work (six out of ten compared with nine out of ten). Fathers in the UK, like other men in the UK generally, work long hours, and longer hours than those in other European countries. Sole-earner fathers work even longer hours still, with evening and weekend work commonplace.

The employment of mothers with dependent children has increased from just under a half in 1973 to six in ten in 1995 and dual-earner families are now the norm among couples with children, but fathers' earnings still account for the bulk of family income. Mothers are still more likely to work part time.

A study of 6000 mothers and fathers aged 33 (Ferri and Smith, 1996) confirms these general findings. Four per cent of this sample were in households with no earner and these households suffered severe economic disadvantage. These disadvantages affected a disproportionately large number of children as these families tended to be the largest, with 22% of the mothers having four or more children.

Fathers and family life

It is difficult to know whether fathers are spending more time caring for their children or not because there is very little earlier evidence with which to compare current information. Ferri and Smith (1996) compared information from the NCDS of 1965 and 1991 which showed, in both years, half of the fathers described as playing an equal part in caring for their children. There is evidence that both mothers and fathers are spending more time on childcare (Gershuny, 1996), but whatever the increase in the caring role of fathers, mothers remain responsible for organising it. General themes emerging from the research on families (Burghes *et al.*, 1997) indicate that families still spend time on shared activities, and that there has been a small increase in the sharing of domestic chores between mothers and fathers, but in general women spend more time on childcare than men and are largely responsible for the core domestic chores, even when they work full time and even when fathers are unemployed.

North American studies have similarly found that fathers spend much less time with their children than mothers and that maternal employment does not lead to fathers assuming more responsibility for such things as the care of sick children, management and selection of child care, or being available at short notice (Lamb, 1997). Men regularly indicate that workplace practices are one of the most important barriers to their greater involvement in caring for children, but men do not trade work time for family time in the same way as women – women translate each hour not spent in paid work into 40–45 minutes of family work compared with men who translate each hour into only 20 minutes (Pleck, 1983).

The research by Nobes and Smith (2000) indicates that fathers read to their children less than mothers and are less intimate with them. This study found significant levels of association between mothers' and fathers' use of physical punishments, indicating that if one parent physically punishes frequently or severely, the other parent is also likely to do so. These findings demonstrate the importance of taking into account both parents' punishments of children when measuring the extent to which children are physically punished (Nobes and Smith, 1997). There are consistent findings that fathers specialise in playing with their children, but it is important to remember that in absolute terms mothers play with their children more than fathers do, even though a greater proportion of the time fathers spend with their children is spent in play (Lamb, 1997). A study looking specifically at fathers and adolescents suggests that a distinction should be made between distance and detachment. This study found that fathers had less involvement than mothers with children overall, but equal involvement when it came to studies or discipline. It also found that fathers' inclination to be distant can allow them to be more capable than mothers of acceptance and respect for an adolescent's wish to be separate (Shulman and Seiffge-Krenke, 1996).

Summary points on the context of fatherhood

- The dominant image to emerge from the socio-demographic picture is that most fathers live with their children and with the child's mother.

- Family type varies depending on the age of the head of the family, social class, geographical location and ethnicity of the family.

- Over half of the women and nearly half the men in Britain do not support the traditional breadwinning model of fatherhood, but the empirical evidence suggests that fathers are still the main earners in families.

- The unemployment rate for young fathers is very high, making it impossible for them to play a breadwinning role.

- For resident fathers in general the employment rates are high. Fathers in employment work long hours and sole earners work even longer.

- There has been a small increase in the domestic tasks undertaken by men but mothers remain primarily responsible for the core domestic tasks.

- Children are disproportionately affected by the severe economic disadvantages common in households with no wage earner because these households tend to have a larger number of children.

Chapter 3

Context: The legal framework

In complex family situations, the legal status of men connected with children, inside or outside the home, can be unclear.

Married men

When a child is born to a married couple the law assumes that the husband is the father of the child. Fathers who are, or were, married to the child's mother at the time of the child's birth share parental responsibility (see below) with the mother.

Unmarried fathers

Biological fathers not married to the child's mother are defined as parents by the *Children Act 1989*. They do not automatically have parental responsibility but they can acquire it by agreement with the mother or by court order (Section 4(1) *Children Act 1989*). The number of parental responsibility agreements and orders made in 1999 was 10 199 (Court Service, 2000). It is likely that changes to the law in the near future will give non-married fathers automatic parental responsibility with certain exceptions, for example to cover situations where the child is born as a result of rape.

Parental responsibility

The definition of parental responsibility in the *Children Act 1989* refers to 'all the rights, duties, powers, responsibilities and authority which by law a parent of the child has in relation to the child and his property'. Practically, having parental responsibility means being able to make decisions about the day-to-day life of a child, for example where the child should go to school or whether or not the child should have medical treatment. The issue of whether or not a father has parental responsibility becomes significant when there is conflict within the family itself or when the state intervenes in the family's life.

Accommodation

Thus, only those with parental responsibility can consent to children being accommodated under Section 20 of the *Children Act 1989* and only those with parental responsibility can remove children from such accommodation.

Care proceedings

If care proceedings are started, while fathers with parental responsibility will automatically be a party to the proceedings, fathers without parental responsibility must be served with notice that the proceedings are being taken and can apply to be a party.

Looked after children

Whether or not fathers have parental responsibility, because they are parents they must be consulted by the local authority who is looking after their child, contact between them and their children should be promoted providing that is consistent with the child's welfare and they have the right to apply to the court for contact with their absent child.

Adoption

Only fathers with parental responsibility are entitled to give or withhold consent to a child's adoption. The making of an adoption order in favour of a man, single or married, will give that man parental responsibility for the child.

Residence orders

If a residence order has been made in relation to a child, the person or the people in whose favour the order has been made will have parental responsibility for him or her. Thus, the existence of a residence order limits the extent to which a father with parental responsibility can exercise his rights and responsibilities if the order has not been made in his favour.

Guardianship

It is possible for men to have parental responsibility by virtue of becoming the child's guardian (Section 5 *Children Act 1989*). A guardian can be appointed for a child where the child has no parent with parental responsibility, or in circumstances where a parent who has a residence order in his or her favour has died. In such circumstances the court could, for example, appoint a male family friend, a male relative or the mother's cohabitant. A mother who has sole parental responsibility for her child can appoint a guardian in her will.

Non-molestation and exclusion orders

The *Family Law Act 1996* Part IV (Family Homes and Domestic Violence) came into force on 1 October 1997. It provides a unified framework for regulating the occupation of a home and for the protection of children and adults from domestic violence or molestation. Women can apply for non-molestation orders to protect themselves and/or their children against their husbands and partners or former husbands and partners. They may also seek exclusion orders against them, the object of such an order being to exclude the man from the home and/or from a defined area around the home. An emergency protection order or interim care order in relation to a child can have an exclusion requirement attached to it. If a non-molestation order or exclusion order is in force against a father or father figure this will necessarily impact on his role within the family.

Stepfathers

Men may be described as stepfathers whether or not they are married to the child's mother, whether or not they are still married and whether or not they live with the child. Alternatively, they may be described as the mother's current or former partner, cohabitee or boyfriend. The use of the term 'stepfather' suggests a closer connection with any children in the family than 'boyfriend' or 'cohabitee'. The situation is made more complex by the fact that different people use these words to mean different things.

The National Stepfamily Association defines a stepfamily as:

> A step-family is created when someone who is already a parent forms a relationship with a new partner who then becomes a step-parent to the children. In some step-families both partners have children who then become stepbrothers and sisters. They may not all live in the same household, but some with their other parent, creating both a full time and a part time step-family household. All the children who have connections with the parent and step-parent belong to the step-family and the structure may involve two step-parents if both birth parents have formed new partnerships (Batchelor *et al.*, 1994).

Stepfathers may or may not have parental responsibility in relation to their stepchildren. They will have parental responsibility if a residence order has been made in favour of the children's mother and the stepfather jointly, or if there has been a step-parent adoption. If neither of these orders has been made they will not have parental responsibility and will not, by law, be a parent, but they will be a relative of the child. Both the *Children Act 1989* and *Family Law Act 1996* include stepparents and stepchildren in their definition of relatives. The *Family Law Act* defines cohabitants as a man and a woman who, although not married to each other, are living together as husband and wife (Section 62 (1)).

Comment

How a father actually relates to his children will have more to do with the practicalities of the family's life than his legal status. A father who is the child's parent may be living with the mother or outside the home. Wherever he lives, he may be very involved in the care and upbringing of the child or he may not. He may be having contact with his child or he may not. It is important is to find out the nature of the relationship between the father figure and the children, and the role the man takes in relation to these children.

Chapter 4

Context: Fathers in families involved in the child protection process

In looking at the information that exists on fathers and families in the studies disseminated through *Child Protection: messages from research*, it is important to bear in mind the following.

- The studies were not specifically looking for information on fathers or father figures. Detailed information on them is limited in comparison with the information available on fathers generally which is referred to in Chapter 3.
- The studies were all of families involved in the child protection process but at different points in that process. The exceptions to this are the two normative studies looking at normal family sexuality and parental control within the family (Nobes and Smith, 2000). Details of the studies are in the Appendix. Cleaver and Freeman (1995) were looking at a sample of families where there were concerns or suspicions of child maltreatment. In some of these families no action was taken beyond an initial enquiry. Sharland *et al.* (1995) were looking at cases at the same threshold point but these were only referrals concerning suspected child sexual abuse. Gibbons *et al.* (1995a) tracked all referrals coming into the child protection process. Thoburn *et al.* (1995) looked at a sample of children and families where

the children had been the subject of a child protection conference and where about half of the children had their names added to the Child Protection Register. Pitcairn *et al.* (1993) had a similar sample group. Farmer and Owen (1995) looked at a sample of families where the children had been the subject of a child protection conference and their names had been placed on the register. Gibbons *et al.* (1995b) followed up children ten years on from their names being placed on a register and compared these children with a similar group of children who had not been through the process.

- The fathers or father figures from which this research evidence comes are thus from families where there are concerns, sometimes very serious, about the wellbeing of the children in those families.

- Within this group there are fathers and father figures who are responsible for the harm done to their children and others who are not; there are differences in the nature of the harm caused; there are men who are violent and/or aggressive and others who are not; and there are those with a high level of needs of their own and others who are functioning well.

- Although the research focuses on a particular group of fathers, the examples of practice in providing services for or working with fathers covers a wider range, extending to fathers of children in need generally.

- One of the key messages from the studies disseminated in *Messages from Research* is that multi-agency cooperation in the provision of services to children and families is as important as cooperation in child protection enquiries and processes. Other commentators have noted that it is not only social workers who fail to engage fathers: health and education professionals do the same (Marsh, 1987; Brown, 1982; Jackson, 1984). The messages about working with fathers and father figures of children in need apply, therefore, to all professionals working with children and families, not just to those working in the sphere of social care.

Children in need: child protection

The *Children Act 1989* places a general duty on local authorities to safeguard and promote the welfare of children in need in their area and to promote their upbringing by their families, as long as this is consistent with their welfare. In order to do so, local authorities should identify the extent to which there are children in need within their area, provide an appropriate range and level of services, and publish their plans for the provision of services (Section 17 and Schedule 2).

The term 'in need' is defined in the Act. There are three elements to the definition:

a   *the child is unlikely to achieve or maintain, or have the opportunity of achieving or maintaining, a reasonable standard of health or development without the provision of services by a local authority; or*

b   *the child's health or development is likely to be significantly impaired, or further impaired, without provision for the child of such services; or*

c   *the child is disabled* (Section 17(10)).

Local authorities also have specific duties to prevent children in their area from suffering neglect or abuse (Schedule 2, para 4) and when they have reasonable cause to suspect that a child in their area is suffering or is likely to suffer significant harm, to make enquiries to enable them to decide what action, if any, is necessary to safeguard the child's welfare (Section 47). 'Harm' covers physical and sexual abuse, the impairment of physical, intellectual, social or behavioural development, and mental and physical health. The process for carrying out these enquiries is not set out in legislation but in detailed government guidance (Department of Health *et al.*, 1999).

Child Protection: messages from research showed that 160 000 initial enquiries were carried out each year in England. The family was visited in about 120 000 cases. There were around 40 000 initial child protection conferences each year and around 24 500 new additions to the Child Protection Register each year. A very small number of children were removed from home in an emergency (around 1500), and many of these returned home quickly. However, it is not clear how many children in England and Wales come within the definition of 'in need' to whom local authorities owe a duty to provide services. It is estimated that between 300 000–400 000 children are in need in England at any one time (Department of Health *et al.*, 2000). A key message from *Messages from Research* was that children in need of protection are also children in need.

The number of children whose names were on the Child Protection Register at 31 March 1999 was 31 900 (Department of Health, 1999). Most of these children remain living at home without any legal action being taken in relation to them. Of the children who started to be looked after during the 1998/9 year, 4700 (17%) were accommodated compulsorily (Department of Health, 2000a). Roughly a third of these children started to be looked after under police protection, a third under emergency protection orders and a third were on remand, committed for trial or detained. During 1998 6017 care orders were made as were 829 supervision orders (Department of Health, 2000b).

Specifically with regard to the role of fathers or father figures in this process, they may come into contact with childcare practitioners because they have children in need and they are seeking and/or receiving services as a result. In certain cases, issues may emerge that lead to child protection procedures being instituted. Other fathers or father figures may have their first contact with practitioners as a result of child protection enquiries.

Family structure

Considering the child protection studies as a whole produces a composite finding that at the time of the initial enquiry only two-fifths (38%) of children whose families enter the child protection process live with both their birth parents – in other words, a much lower proportion than the national average of around 73%. Around 31% live with a lone mother and 28%

in reconstituted families, a higher proportion than the national averages of 19% and 8% respectively. A small proportion, probably about 2%, and certainly no more than 4%, reside with a lone father, which is the same as the national average.

Fathers' involvement in the households fluctuates. More fathers are living at home at the start of enquiries than later. Early on in the process of the child protection enquiry, a number of fathers leave for a variety of reasons, so that immediately after the initial child protection conference the number of children living with both parents has fallen to 26% (Thoburn *et al.*, 1995; Farmer and Owen, 1995). By later stages in the process, many of these remaining men had left. Gibbons *et al.* (1995b) found that less than a fifth (17%) of the 144 children followed up ten years after their names were added to the Child Protection Register were living with the same two parents as at the time of registration. Three-quarters were still living with one of their original carers but a fifth of fathers had left the household and many had been replaced by a new man.

What about non-resident fathers? Thoburn *et al.* (1995) identified 68 in their study of 220 cases; 52 fathers and 16 stepfathers. The research team separated the cases into three groups. First, there were men who left home at the time the abuse enquiry began. Some of these departed because they were implicated in the enquiry, but Cleaver and Freeman (1995) and Sharland *et al.* (1995) remind us that the stress experienced by families as a result of being the subject of child protection enquiries can be a cause of parental discord and even breakdown. Second, there were men who had previously left the household and were implicated in the current enquiry. Finally, there were men who had previously left the household and were not in any way implicated.

Stressors

The evidence about fathers living in these households paints a picture of multiple, often interacting, stressors. Gibbons *et al.* (1995a) notes that three-fifths (57%) of the households

they studied lacked a wage earner and, in two-parent households, two-fifths of the father figures were unemployed.
Pitcairn *et al.* (1993) found that 83% of mothers and 75% of
fathers were unemployed. The other studies show similarly
high levels of unemployment and dependency on state
benefits. High levels of income support indicated considerable
poverty.

In over a quarter (27%) of cases, domestic violence was
found to be a feature at the start of the enquiry. This was
established from case files or from other information obtained
during the previous five years if the family were already
known to social services (Gibbons, 1995a). Information
collected at subsequent stages such as child protection conferences or registration shows even higher levels of domestic
violence (*see* page 46). There were high levels (35%) of
domestic discord (Thoburn *et al.*, 1995), and a small but
significant number of fathers had criminal records, histories
of mental health problems, substance misuse and/or abuse in
their own childhoods (*see* page 45 for more details). Irrespec-
tive of whether they were maltreating their children, these
fathers were struggling to support them.

Fathers as perpetrators

The studies give details of the reasons for the child's name being
placed on the Child Protection Register, including the type of
maltreatment suffered and the relationship of the known or
alleged perpetrator. Such figures can give some information
about fathers or father figures as perpetrators but they are not
prevalence figures. In addition, it needs to be borne in mind
that the process of registration itself is gender-biased so that
more cases of abuse by mothers are registered than cases of
abuse by fathers (*see* page 27 and Farmer and Owen, 1998).

Gibbons *et al.* (1995b) found that in two-fifths (43%) of
cases where the child's name had been placed on the Child
Protection Register the harm could be attributed to a male
care giver, which indicates that in three-fifths of cases the
responsibility lay elsewhere. In 40% of cases, the female care

giver was responsible and in another 11%, both male and female care givers were involved. The other studies show similar proportions: fathers or father figures were either solely or jointly responsible in 36% of cases (Farmer and Owen, 1995); in 36% (Cleaver and Freeman, 1995); in 55% (Thoburn *et al.*, 1995); and mothers in 36% (Farmer and Owen, 1995); in 40% (Cleaver and Freeman, 1995); and in 45% (Thoburn *et al.*, 1995). In a subsequent study by Thoburn *et al.* (2000) which looked only at children whom practitioners and researchers identified as suffering or likely to suffer significant harm, mothers were responsible in 61% of cases and fathers or father figures in 28%. In this latter study, a higher proportion of the children, as compared with those in the earlier study, were living with a lone mother (43%). This is hardly surprising as adults living with the child have the most opportunity to harm them, but these figures indicate that fathers and father figures are a greater risk to children than mothers if one takes into account the fact that, compared with fathers, mothers are more likely to be the primary carers.

There is variation in the involvement of fathers in situations where children are harmed – both by type of household and type of harm. In reconstituted families, the father is 50% solely or partly responsible for the harm, compared with 37% in families where both parents are present. The following table from Gibbons *et al.* (1995b) illustrates this point.

Perpetrator	Lone %	Type of household		Other %	All %
		Joint %	Recon-stituted %		
Female parent/substitute	65	24	28	0	34
Male parent/substitute	19	37	50	25	37
Both/either	5	10	11	25	10
Other	3	6	4	50	5
No injury	8	23	7	0	14

N=165 (5 missing data).

This highlights the importance of research studies that distinguish fathers from father figures and are specific about the nature and severity of the maltreatment (Sternberg, 1997). The type of harm caused by fathers also differs. Farmer and Owen (1995) found that 15 (34%) of their 44 cases concerned sexual abuse; all the perpetrators were male and over half were fathers or father figures. In the 16 cases (36%) of physical abuse, mothers were responsible in seven cases and fathers or father figures in six. In neglect and emotional abuse cases the mother was regarded as mainly responsible. The Sharland *et al.* study (1995), looking only at referrals for suspected sexual abuse, found that in their sample of 220 cases, birth fathers were suspected of responsibility in 28% of cases, father figures in 16% and known but unrelated male adults in 32%.

Action taken

From what is reported in the Department of Health studies, it is clear that the presence or absence of fathers in the household makes a difference to the way enquiries progress, at least in the short term. Gibbons *et al.* (1995a) identified a number of different factors that were associated with children being filtered out of the child protection process early on and these included cases where there was no man in the household (especially not a stepfather figure), the alleged perpetrator was not in the household, or where the referral concerned neglect or emotional abuse rather than physical or sexual abuse. The studies indicate that fathers and father figures are more likely to be perpetrators in sexual abuse cases and as likely as mothers to be perpetrators in physical abuse cases (see above). Cases filtered out prior to a child protection conference included those where there were only girls in the household, where the perpetrator was not in the household or where no parent figure was recorded as having a criminal record, a history of substance misuse, a psychiatric disorder, a history of domestic violence or having been abused as a child (Gibbons *et al.*, 1995a).

Action to get the perpetrator to leave home was more common in cases of child sexual abuse than in other categories of maltreatment and in these situations it was rare for the perpetrator and the child not to be separated. The Farmer and Owen (1995) study shows that in the cases of child sexual abuse, 60% of abusers and 40% of the children left the home and in only two cases did the child remain at home with the abuser. In contrast, where physical abuse had occurred only 25% of those responsible for the harm left home and 56% of children (nine) remained living with the perpetrator. Farmer and Owen also found that when the person responsible for the harm was thought to be a man, it was more likely that action would be taken to remove him, whereas when it was a woman there was more likelihood of the child being removed.

Farmer and Owen's study found that when mothers, rather than fathers or male partners, were considered responsible for abuse or neglect, the child's name was much more likely to be placed on the Child Protection Register. Thus the child was registered in 78% of cases where the mother was held responsible (55% natural fathers; 60% stepfathers). The difference was greater still in cases of physical abuse. The children of over three-quarters (77%) of physically abusing mothers were registered, compared with fewer than half (48%) of the children of physically abusing fathers (*see also* Burgess, 1997, for a discussion of gender bias in the child protection system).

Summary points

- The structure of families involved in the child protection process at any stage is different from the general socio-demographic picture in that fewer children live with both their own parents (38% as opposed to 70%) and more live with lone parents (31%) or in reconstituted families (28%).

- There are high levels of unemployment and poverty – 57% of households referred into the child protection system lacked a wage earner.

- There are high levels of domestic violence (27% recorded at the time of referral and higher levels at subsequent stages) and partner discord (35%).

- A small but significant number of fathers had a criminal record or experienced mental or physical health problems, were substance misusers or had experienced abuse in their own childhoods.

- Fathers and father figures are a greater risk to children than mothers if you take into account the fact that mothers are more often the primary carers for children. However, more evidence is necessary regarding the maltreatment of children which distinguishes between fathers and father figures as perpetrators.

- In reconstituted families, it is more likely that the father figure will be solely or partly responsible for the harm.

- The information obtained from child protection registers on those who cause harm to children indicates that there is a difference between the type of harm caused by fathers and father figures and by mothers. Fathers and father figures are responsible exclusively for sexual abuse and as responsible as mothers for physical abuse. It is important to remember that the process of registration is itself gender-biased.

- Gender bias operates in the child protection system in that it is more likely that a child's name will be placed on the Child Protection Register if the mother is responsible for the maltreatment – either because she is the sole carer or because professionals regard her as the main carer.

Chapter 5

Messages from Research

Child Protection: messages from research (1995a) identified five preconditions of effective practice to safeguard children and promote their welfare. These were:

- sensitive and informed professional–client relationships
- an appropriate balance of power between participants
- a wide perspective on child protection
- effective supervision and training of social workers
- services which enhance children's general quality of life.

The studies indicate that if these conditions prevail, outcomes for children in terms of their overall welfare are generally better. These five conditions are also relevant when considering how professionals can work best with the fathers in children's lives, to ensure the child's protection and the promotion of his or her welfare.

Sensitive and informed professional–client relationships

Ask, don't assume

It is clear from the accumulated evidence that professionals have to display great sensitivity when dealing with gender issues within families. Taking into account the family's culture, class and ethnicity is recognised as a priority consideration in social work, even though there is sometimes a gap between aspiration and practice. But, when it comes to the particular task of testing assumptions about the role of fathers or of the man in the family, whether he lives in the home or outside it, then it appears that such sensitivity is less marked.

The 'culture' within the family can relate as much to socio-economic as to ethnic background. The case studies in the research demonstrate by the variety of situations they describe, for example, that it is not justifiable to assume that in this particular family from this particular socioeconomic group or in this family from this particular ethnic background, men would not be expected to share in childcare tasks. It is important to ask family members what happens in their family. Similarly, it is not wise to take for granted what women in the families think men should be doing. Women may want their husband, partner or former partner to be more involved in looking after the children or in dealing with welfare agencies and it may be the men who back away from closer involvement. On the other hand, women may feel that men have no part to play in childcare or in dealing with welfare agencies. They may fear that involving men in these areas of life will undermine their own role.

Surveys in the USA which show that a majority of men want to be more involved with their children also indicate that the majority of women do not want their husbands to be more involved than they currently are (Pleck, 1982; Quinn and Staines, 1979). Other research suggests that, within individual families, agreement between mothers and fathers regarding paternal roles is more important than what those roles are, because fundamental conflicts between parents have adverse effects on children's development. It is important to distinguish between families where the father is highly involved because that is what the parents want from those where the father is involved merely because he is unemployed. Both parents may be very unhappy with the latter situation, so provoking conflict that has a negative impact on the children (Lamb, 1997). *Life on a Low Income* describes vividly the feeling of worthlessness experienced by unemployed men because they are no longer the breadwinner (Kempson, 1996).

If professionals are sure that a child's welfare will be promoted and enhanced by direct work with the father figure, on his own or as part of joint work with the family, they should explain to the woman and the man what work could be undertaken and how it would benefit the child. In some instances, direct work with the family will involve helping the members discuss and define their roles. This can be particularly helpful if the father or father figure has become unemployed. If a father or father figure is to remain in the home but there are concerns about him, for example because he is known to have physically abused children in the past, the practitioner can help the parents negotiate and specify their roles – so that, in this example, the father or father figure would not be involved in disciplining the children or could be helped to find new ways of managing the children's behaviour.

Working in partnership with families involves respecting the family's way of doing things, but sometimes it will emerge that the family's way of doing things is aggravating the problems and change is needed. Burgess and Ruxton (1996) argue that workers impose their values on families in any event, and that they should be prepared to question the traditional assumptions of some of the families they work with.

Clarify relationships

When becoming involved with a family or undertaking an enquiry, professionals should ask a number of questions about fathers and about men living in the home. First, is the father living in the house or out of it? Second, if he is living in the house, what is his relationship with the other carer (if there is one) and child? Is he the birth father or has he adopted a father's role in relation to the children? What is his legal status, if any, in relation to the children? Third, if he is out of the home, what is his involvement in the child's life, legally, financially and emotionally? Principal questions here will be about past and current contact with the children and future intentions to maintain or resurrect family links. Fourth, are there known factors present that may affect a father's ability to safeguard or promote his children's welfare, such as poverty, poor housing, learning disabilities, physical or mental illness, domestic violence, alcohol or drug misuse, and the father's own childhood experiences? Finally, in some cases, there will be a question of possible or actual harm to a child or a mother and the father's role in that. These questions are summarised in Figure 1.

Generally, both in the professional world and that of research, there are missing data on many of the dimensions shown in Figure 1. Routinely assembling a thorough family history on all children would remedy the situation but not without raising issues for practitioners about whom they should collect their information from. Ideally the fathers and father figures should be spoken to directly, but in some circumstances mothers will be reluctant to disclose details about non-resident fathers and the situation will need to be handled sensitively. Thoburn *et al.* (1995) note in their study that there were hardly any social or family histories on the files that were written specifically as family histories as opposed to being prepared at a later date for court proceedings or child protection conferences. However, it seems clear that if this information were to be collected and recorded fully and accurately on the files, then practitioners, researchers and, most importantly, families would benefit (Department of Health *et al.*, 2000).

Guidance on working in partnership with families involved in the child protection process emphasises the importance of involving fathers and father figures directly in the enquiries.

It is routine practice to see a child's mother. It should be equally standard practice to see relevant adult males, both those in the household and those living elsewhere who have parental responsibility. This is essential because they are part of the child's life and are significant either for positive or negative reasons. If professionals aspire to partnership with parents and carers it is a poor beginning to undervalue the contributions of men known to the child. Such an approach may be based on assumptions of guilt or

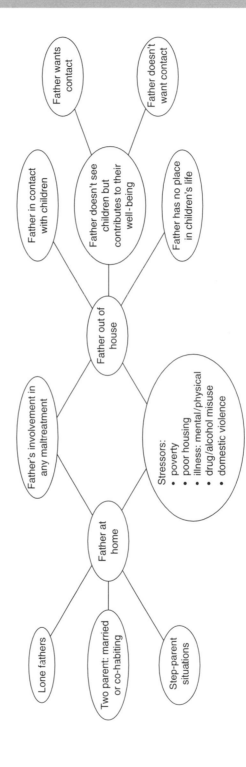

Figure 1 Father's role in possible or actual harm to a child or a mother.

insignificance which prove unfounded when the situation is explored properly. It may also be dangerous for the child if the worker makes only a second-hand assessment of a man's potential to protect or abuse the child in the future. Additionally such action may collude with any wish the alleged abuser may have to deny involvement in the abuse (Department of Health, 1995b).

Non-resident fathers

The studies show that while some fathers and stepfathers will leave the home because they have harmed or abused a child, others will have had no involvement in the child's maltreatment. Some out-of-home fathers were in contact with their children, others were not. Non-resident fathers who had been away for some time and were not in contact with their children were rarely involved in the child protection enquiries or assessments or invited to child protection conferences. The same was also true of fathers who had maintained contact with their children. Not only were they not involved, they were not always informed of what was happening. Thoburn *et al.* give this example of missing information (1995, p 62).

> Three boys were removed from their mother's care when one told a casualty officer that the serious burn on his arm had been deliberately inflicted by his mother with an iron. The father was a caring parent in regular contact with his sons, aware of the stresses within the family, and wanting to do all he could to support the children remaining with their mother. He was not present at the child protection conference, but was subsequently contacted when the children were in care.

> In another case a non-resident father was accused by his ex-wife of hitting their four-year-old so hard on his bottom that it left a bruise. The child regularly stayed with his father to give the mother a break. The father denied the allegation when interviewed by the police. The father was not invited to the child protection conference, which the mother

attended. The father received a letter two months later telling him what the results of the conference were. The social worker had no direct contact with the father other than a phone call. During the research interview the worker said that on reflection he thought it would have been useful to have involved the father at an earlier stage as he would have learned more about the family which might have been helpful in the provision of longer-term support.

The research for these studies took place before the implementation of the *Children Act 1989* and it would be interesting to see whether the stress on the importance of the wider family in legislation has led to changes in practice.

Thoburn *et al.* (1995) and Farmer and Owen (1995) give examples of the positive roles that non-resident fathers can play.

Jonathan, a seven-year-old boy who was beaten by his mother's cohabitee, went to live with his father. He was in the group of children who had the best outcomes; that is the child was not only protected but his welfare was enhanced and the needs of his parents were met. In Jonathan's case, the successful placement was not consequent to the social worker's plan. His father simply stepped in to fill an obvious need once the boy's name had been placed on the Child Protection Register. The shock of social work involvement had called forth increased resources from within the extended family (Farmer and Owen, 1995, pp 293–5).

Patsy was the two-year-old daughter of a young mother whose problems in coping had started soon after Patsy's father had left home. The concerns were around rubbish and dirt in the house and garden and general neglect of Patsy, who was dirty, underfed and inappropriately dressed for the weather. Apart from some delay with speech, she was physically fit, developing well and very attached to her mother. There was social work involvement over a period of time to try and improve the general level of care, but eventually a child protection conference was held and Patsy was registered. Over the next year, Patsy's mother was still finding it difficult to cope and Patsy was looked after under voluntary arrangements on three occasions. Her father discovered this via local rumour on the third occasion. He had been in regular contact with Patsy until six months before the first conference. He had stopped visiting because of the rows the visits caused. He had also moved house. When he heard what was happening he contacted social services straight away. He was angry and upset that he had not known what was going on. He would willingly have had Patsy to stay with him and his new partner and her children if he had been asked. Once he became involved, the parents were able to work out a satisfactory arrangement for shared care. As a result of his involvement a less intensive protection plan was agreed with Patsy's mother (Thoburn *et al.*, 1995, p 46).

This study by Thoburn *et al.* looked at the nature and extent of family involvement in the child protection process and found that at the enquiry stage, 40% of non-resident fathers were rated by the researchers as not involved or as being placated or manipulated by professionals at this stage, as opposed to 7% of main carers. At the point of the child protection plan being made, non-resident parents were least likely to be involved. The rating of agency and social work practice with non-resident parents indicated that it was likely to result in their involvement in only about one-third of cases. But 'in some cases social workers went to considerable lengths, even when there were no agency policies about the involvement of a non-resident parent, to make sure they were fully informed and were enabled to attend child protection and other meetings' (p 180).

Information

Families are entitled to information about the social work process, the purpose of any intervention and their rights in relation to it; they may also benefit from a range of other information depending on the nature of their problems and how they themselves identify their needs. This could include information on welfare rights, benefits, housing, childcare, specialist health, education, alcohol and drugs services, practical help and legal remedies in relation to domestic violence, disputes over children and divorce, and details of relevant local or community groups. Department of Health guidance stresses the importance of families receiving full information in all circumstances (Department of Health, 1995b).

Professionals require information about the family history, family structure, extended family, legal status of family members, the family's perception of its problems, and the family's views about the roles of men and women in caring for children in order to intervene appropriately. Bearing in mind the findings of the Thomas Coram Research Unit (Nobes and Smith, 1997; 2000; and *see* page 10) information on levels and types of punishment used by both mothers and fathers and father figures is also important. In addition, guidance on working with children experiencing domestic violence states 'there is evidence to suggest that good practice consists of asking **all** women routinely about domestic violence in **every** case. The very fact of asking about domestic violence conveys an important message to women and children that practitioners are aware of its existence and relevance, thus possibly facilitating disclosure' (Hester *et al.*, 1998).

Difficulties in practice

The development of sensitive and informed client–professional relationships is clearly an essential part of working in partnership with children and their families. However, with respect to fathers involved in child protection enquiries, such an aim can be difficult to achieve. The studies have examples of fathers who distance themselves from the process and from practitioners – who, on occcasions, may unconsciously collude because they are more at ease working with mothers. Fathers may show hostility towards practitioners or their violent behaviour may undermine the mother's ability to cooperate.

An insensitive approach or response to a mother may drive her to side with a father whose behaviour is the cause of concern. For a more detailed discussion of the ways in which men are avoided by practitioners working in social care with children and families see O'Hagan and Dillenburger (1995).

Summary points

- Professionals should 'ask and not assume' what role the father(s) and any father figures play in the family.

- Collecting information on the family's circumstances should be done routinely. This should include information about the fathers and/or father figures, whether they are resident in the home and under what circumstances.

- Fathers should be involved in discussions about the child's welfare and in any therapeutic work (whilst ensuring the child's safety).

- If the father is absent from the home, establish his involvement in the child's life – emotionally, legally and financially – and what contact he has with his children.

- As well as collecting information from families, including fathers, professionals should give families information. If direct work with fathers is planned, explain to all family members the purpose of this work.

Achieving the right balance of power between professionals, parents and other relatives and children

Responding to the mother's concerns

The importance of achieving the right balance of power applies to relationships within the family as well as to relationships between professionals and the family. The studies show that just under half of all referrals in the various samples came from the family itself – around 20% from mothers, 15% from children (often disclosing abuse to their mothers or friends), another 10% from other family members, including 3% from fathers. The professional groups who came closest to this were teachers (15%) and health professionals (12%) (Thoburn *et al.*, 1995; Cleaver and Freeman, 1995).

Several of the research studies (Farmer and Owen, 1995; Cleaver and Freeman, 1995; Thoburn *et al.*, 1995; Sharland *et al.*, 1995) found that many of the mothers who expressed concerns to professionals or reported injuries did so because they were hoping for advice and help themselves, and also for assistance in regulating the actions of the men with whom they were living, often because of violence. But, when child protection procedures were initiated, these were viewed unsympathetically by mothers who felt betrayed, undermined and disempowered: they felt angry, distrustful and unwilling to accept help in the future. Lack of support meant that some women formed alliances against external agencies with their male partner, who had harmed the child.

Other mothers, by contrast, were unwilling to express concerns about the behaviour of the men in their families out of fear that they would lose their children as a result of revealing domestic violence or drug or alcohol misuse. Professionals were, in many cases, unaware of the existence of these problems (Farmer and Owen, 1995, p 79).

The studies found that although couples frequently showed an outwardly united front to professionals, inside the home it could be a very different story. Many mothers were far more concerned about the behaviour of their partners than they publicly acknowledged to professionals. In such situations, intervention could lead to increased domestic tensions and even family breakdown. It often resulted in mothers taking *more* responsibility for childcare, some women even giving up work to spend more time at home. It was mothers who felt the burden of protecting children from further harm.

Exclusive focus on mothers

The tendency to focus on mothers, regardless of whether they are the source of the family's problems, has already been noted, as has the fact that even where the man living in the home was responsible for the harm to the child, the focus of the professionals quickly shifted to the mother. In some cases, this shift was clearly attributable to the view of fathers adopted by professionals. Where there was to be ongoing involvement with the family, professionals concentrated on working with the mother rather than on the problematic father or the relationship between them. Where concerns about the children related to neglect as opposed to specific abusive incidents, there was often less clarity about which parent was thought to be responsible; but, even then, professional attention still focused on the mother: 'Whether or not the mother was responsible for the abuse, she was usually the person who took responsibility for the child and mediated between her husband and the outside world' (Farmer and Owen, 1995). Farmer and Owen also note that the assessment of risk of harm to the child could be unduly focused on the mother with the danger that social workers actually reinforced a situation in which male abusers found it easy to opt out. Social workers were working with the women when the danger came from the men (p 317).

Guard against blaming mothers

Professional attitudes seem to be more punitive towards mothers who harm their children than towards fathers who harm them. As a consequence, they expect more of mothers and take the harm they cause more seriously. It has already been noted that in the Farmer and Owen study, researchers found a greater tendency to register children in cases where women were responsible for the harm. The researchers wondered whether this is because in two-parent households where the man is causing harm it is assumed that the mother will protect the child, whereas in lone-parent households children may be more vulnerable to registration simply because the majority of lone parents are mothers.

Farmer and Owen found a significant correlation between unfavourable comments made about mothers at initial child protection conferences and a decision to register, but no comparable connection with unfavourable comments about fathers. They also noted that in two-parent households the question of whether the non-abusing parent could protect the child was considered far more in relation to mothers (in 60% of the relevant cases) than in relation to father figures (in 19% of relevant cases).

Researchers were anxious to point out that it is not always appreciated that mothers are placed in a difficult situation when abuse is suspected, whatever the family circumstances. Registration was experienced as an additional burden for women when it was the fathers who had abused. The mothers felt judged and responsible, and fathers sometimes reacted by opting out of the disciplining role completely, so putting still greater pressure on their partners. A similar result was found in earlier studies (Marsh, 1987).

Mothers who were coping with fathers who were uninvolved with their children found that professional involvement tended to encourage that distance, rather than stimulating the fathers to enhance their parenting role. Yet, mothers who were concerned about the way their partners treated their children felt that they were responsible for ensuring their future protection and that they would be blamed if they were unsuccessful. Mothers experiencing domestic violence, or concerned about drug or alcohol misuse by their partner, felt not only fear for their own safety but also anxiety that if anything further happened they might lose their children. Sometimes a mother's failure to cooperate with professionals arose from her fear of the consequences for herself if she did what was being suggested; for example, Cleaver and Freeman describe how one mother refused a nursery place for her child because she feared being beaten up if she accepted it (Cleaver and Freeman, 1995; O'Hagan and Dillenburger, 1995).

When a referral comes from a mother, the challenge for the professionals is to respond to her request for help in a way that addresses the particular problems she has identified, that ensures the child's protection from significant harm in cases where that is an issue, and that does not leave the mother feeling powerless and further undermined at home. When a referral comes from outside the family, professionals should take time to gauge the existing balance of power within the family as the mother's position can be seriously undermined by focusing all attention on her.

Fathers and child protection conferences

The studies found that where both parents were invited to the whole or part of the child protection conference, the majority of the conferences were attended by mothers on their own. But men did attend some, occasionally alone, as the figures in the box below indicate.

Parental attendance at child protection conferences

Parents or other family members were present at 59% of conferences
36 out of 120 (30%) of conferences were attended by mothers only
18 (15%) attended by both parents
4 (3%) attended by mother and stepfather
6 (5%) attended by father on own
2 (1%) attended by fathers and stepmothers
5 (4%) attended by other family members
(Farmer and Owen, 1995, p 108)

Mother and father or male partner attended together in 28 out of 220 conferences (13%)
Father on own attended 4 (2%)
(Thoburn et al., 1995, p 129)

Thoburn *et al.* were surprised that fathers attended as often as they did, especially in light of the often-voiced criticism of social workers' failure to engage men in the process (p 129). Yet, when they did attend, men were generally more active in discussions than women (Farmer and Owen, p 118), which implies that they may be more easily involved in more formal meetings than informal visits to the home. This assumption may perhaps be further strengthened by the fact that research into the use of Family Group Conferences shows that fathers and father figures regularly attend (Marsh and Crow, 1998).

However, the fact that fathers and father figures are often more active in discussions than women is not always a benefit to the child. For example, Farmer and Owen (1995, p 120) describe in detail a child protection conference concerning a 13-year-old girl who had alleged that her stepfather had played with her in a way she found distasteful. The stepfather and the mother were both present at the conference and the stepfather took control of the meeting. The case illustrated that it can be possible for the 'wrong' parent to be empowered if professionals fail to assist parents who are lacking in confidence.

Involve non-resident fathers and other relatives

Sources of support and empowerment are to be found within the wider family, among relatives and some non-resident parents. However, it has already been noted that parents who live separately from the child, whether or not they have been responsible for any harm, were largely excluded from the child protection process. As a consequence, those who were not implicated in harming the child also felt disempowered – they lacked information about what was happening and their views and wishes and feelings were not taken into account.

Involving non-resident fathers in the process requires professionals to make sensitive and rapid judgements about power balances within the family. Mothers may be extremely concerned about the involvement of their former husbands or partners: there may have been domestic violence in the past; men may have maltreated their children; former partners may find out about what is going on within the home; former partners might try and take their children away from them and so on.

Thoburn *et al.* (1995, p 62) give an example of a sensitive approach to a complex case. A mother had three children by three different partners. A child protection conference was held on the youngest child because the father was psychotic and had threatened to kill the baby. The mother had moved away from him. All three fathers were in contact with their children, the last one under supervision. All three fathers were invited to the child protection conference and all attended. Separate waiting areas were arranged for them and they were invited to attend that part of the conference which considered their child, thus preserving confidentiality but allowing maximum participation within the parameters of the confidential information.

The challenge for professionals is to achieve an appropriate balance of power between themselves and the families with whom they are working. In addition, professionals should be encouraged to identify, with the help of family members, the balances of power within the family itself – between partners, between former partners and within the extended family.

Summary points

- Many child protection referrals come from mothers themselves, often because they are seeking help to regulate the behaviour of their partners. However, they can be undermined by the response. They may be viewed unsympathetically and have no control over the chain of events they have set in motion.

- Professionals focus on the mother whether or not she was responsible for the maltreatment.

- Non-resident fathers are minimally involved in the child protection process but the studies contain several examples of how they can, or could, be involved and how they can be a useful resource.

The importance of having a wide perspective

Explore the needs of all family members

A major theme of *Child Protection: messages from research* was professional preoccupation with enquiries, sometimes at the expense of providing effective services. A crude interpretation is that social workers spend a disproportionate amount of time thinking about whether the child has been abused and not enough doing something to help. Thoburn *et al.* (1995) report that the 50% of parents who welcomed professional help, believing it would ease their difficulties, rarely got the services they wanted (pp 144 and 121). Finding out what help a family requires is not straightforward. Often they do not know themselves or they cannot express what they want, or their views differ from those of the professionals. Farmer and Owen (1995) note that parents' needs were not always identified by practitioners. For example, the family's housing situation was mentioned in only 33% of conferences, financial circumstances in 28%, support from the extended family in 36%, other social contacts and support in 18% of conferences.

Identify the specific needs of fathers

Parents of children in need frequently require help because of their own particular problems. This includes fathers. Among a small but significant proportion of fathers in the study by Thoburn *et al.* (1995), there were complicating factors, such as emotional disorders, mental health problems and learning disabilities. They also found a small proportion of men who had an extended history of substance or alcohol abuse, much of it quite serious. Similarly, Farmer and Owen (1995) found that 52% of parents at first interview scored at a level of significant psychological distress. They also found that three of the 14 fathers in their study had sexually assaulted siblings in childhood and one had been sexually abused as a child. Eleven of the men had been seriously physically abused and

two-thirds of them reported damaging experiences of separation and poor relationships with their own parents.

In the study by Pitcairn *et al.* (1993), 60% of the parents
reported having health and emotional problems; 50% of
fathers and 40% of mothers had been in contact with social
workers as a child; 50% of fathers (13% of mothers) had
been to prison or borstal or both; 84% of fathers and 73% of
mothers had no certificate on leaving school; 14% of parents
admitted drug or alcohol problems.

Several of the research teams report considerable discord
between partners. Thoburn *et al.* (1995) record that 17% of
the parents in the sample of 220 cases had previously been or
were presently involved in a custody dispute and there was
evidence of a history of partner conflict in over a third (35%)
of cases. Over half (52%) of parents in Thoburn's study told
of a serious loss by death or divorce of a close relative in the
previous 12 months and a quarter of a serious illness or
accident in the same time period. Sharland *et al.* (1995)
found that 68% of parents had experienced significant difficulties in their lives in the year preceding the referral.
Twenty-five per cent of cases in Thoburn's study involved a
parent or partner who was known to have a history of violent
behaviour. All this has to be viewed in the context of social
isolation; many families in child protection enquiries have
been found to be cut off from their immediate neighbourhood
and commonly used support systems.

Domestic violence was a feature in a significant proportion
of child protection cases. Gibbons *et al.* (1995b) found that at
the point of registration there was evidence of domestic
violence in 51% of the families of the index children. At the
ten-year follow-up stage they found more domestic violence
among the families of the children whose names had been
placed on the register than among the comparison group
families (27% compared with 16%) but it is noteworthy that
the level of domestic violence within the families of the
comparison group is also so high. Where professional and
managerial families are involved in the child protection
process, domestic violence is more likely to be present than

in similar families not involved in the process (22% compared with 10%). Farmer and Owen (1995) found domestic violence in over 50% of their families and it was evident in 20% of cases in the Thoburn study. Research into domestic violence (Mullender and Morley, 1994; Brandon and Lewis, 1996; Hester *et al.*, 1998) shows a connection between domestic violence and the abuse of children. In addition, the effects on children of witnessing domestic violence are now recognised, although this is an area where more research is needed (Sternberg, 1997). Skuse *et al.* (1998), in a study designed to identify the factors that may increase the risk of adolescent boys who had been sexually abused becoming abusers themselves, found that the three most significant factors were exposure to intrafamilial violence, witnessing such violence and discontinuity of care.

Provision of services

Failing to understand the complexity of problems and issues results in a lack of appropriate service provision. Thoburn *et al.* (1995) estimate that less than a fifth (19%) of families were provided with a service appropriate to their identified needs. All the researchers comment on the lack of psychiatric help available in the range of services offered. Farmer and Owen (1995) note that the lack of recognition of needs in relation to domestic violence and substance misuse meant that practitioners failed to engage disaffected parents. It also meant that interventions were unfocused and were not specifically aimed at addressing stressor factors in the family. Supportive social work did little to address these very specific problems.

Summary points

- The inter-relationship and complexity of the needs within families, part of which may be the father's behaviour, should be addressed systematically. As Farmer and Owen (1995) say, a failure to look into the causes of a child's problems and to carry out interventions aimed at alleviating their difficulty leads to a style of social work which, in the end, achieves few of its stated aims and seldom addresses men's problems.

- Men's problems should be looked at separately from those of other family members. The emphasis since the publication of *Child Protection: messages from research* has been on the needs of each child, the assessment of which should extend to fathers' parenting capacity; and fathers' own needs and how these can be met, in the interests of the child and any future children he may have.

- An assessment of the needs of family members is likely to reveal a plethora of difficulties. The research identified a range of problems including those in relation to emotional and physical health, drug and alcohol misuse, marital discord and domestic violence, poverty and poor housing.

Supervision and training of social workers

Practice issues – working in partnership

A key underlying theme of the *Children Act 1989* is that, wherever possible, practitioners should strive to work in partnership with children and families. One of the findings of the *Messages from Research* studies was that where it was possible to work in partnership with the family this led to better outcomes in terms of the children's overall welfare and development.

The study by Thoburn *et al.* (1995) looked specifically at the extent to which professionals were able to work in partnership with those families involved in the child protection process. The definition of partnership that informed the study was that provided by the Family Rights Group (1991) in the Department of Health commissioned training pack

Working in Partnership with Families. Partnership is marked by:

- respect for one another
- rights to information
- accountability
- competence and value accorded to individual input.

In short, each partner is seen as having something to contribute, power is shared, decisions are made jointly, and roles are not only respected but also backed by legal and moral rights (Family Rights Group, 1991).

The Challenge of Partnership in Child Protection: practice guide (Department of Health, 1995b) identifies four approaches to partnership. These are:

- providing information
- involvement
- participation
- partnership (para 2.7).

It is recognised that working in partnership can be particularly difficult to achieve in circumstances where the family's first contact with social workers is because there is concern that the child may be suffering significant harm, or in circumstances where the family disagree with the practitioners' assessment of its presence or likelihood. Working in partnership with fathers and father figures may involve different elements from working in partnership with mothers, depending on the circumstances of the particular child and family. In looking at what makes a family more likely to work in partnership, Thoburn *et al.* (1995) found that the nature of the allegation and the attitudes of family members to that allegation are important. Whereas 57% of parents not responsible for the harm to the child were rated by the researchers as involved in the enquiries and any subsequent intervention, only 33% of those known to have caused harm were. Sharland *et al.* (1995) found that parents faced with an allegation against a member of their family or household were less likely to be able to work in partnership. One of the factors contributing to whether or not professionals could work in partnership with parents was whether or not the alleged abuser accepted a degree of responsibility. Farmer and Owen (1995) found that men accused of sexual abuse hardly ever admitted it and Thoburn *et al.* (1995) found that sexual abuse cases were more likely to come into the 'not involved at all' category.

Thoburn found that where culpability never became clear, those alleged to have caused harm were least likely to participate or be partners, although 11% of them **did** actually become involved. Farmer and Owen (1995) found that where culpability was denied it was difficult for social workers to know where the work should be directed. Lacking concrete evidence, they tended to set up lengthy assessments in the hope that something would emerge.

Thoburn and colleagues found that lone female parents were significantly more likely to participate in working in partnership than either a parenting pair or a lone father. This may well reflect the fact that social workers are able to engage better with women than with men. Although only half as many men as women participated or were partners during the period of the enquiries and the subsequent involvement with the family, a **majority** (65%) did become involved to some extent (Thoburn *et al.*, 1995, pp 191–2).

These findings reflect the difficult nature of the task facing social workers but they may also reflect a failure to engage with difficult men. The task for trainers and supervisers is to encourage practitioners to look for methods of working with fathers responsible, or believed responsible, for harm rather than to assume such work will be impossible. Consideration should perhaps be given more often to allocating a second social worker to work directly with the father. The evidence from the study by Thoburn *et al.* (1995) that a majority of fathers did participate and that there was some participation by sexual abusers indicates there is some scope for improvement. Trainers and supervisors could provide assistance to staff by helping them think about how to disaggregate the parents' needs and in making use of the recording forms which accompany the *Framework for the Assessment of Children in Need and their Families* (Department of Health and Cleaver, 2000; Department of Health *et al.*, 2000) and other guidance such as *The Challenge of Partnership in Child Protection: practice guide* (Department of Health, 1995b).

Family histories

If a detailed family history is not taken, important sources of support and resources within the wider family, including non-resident fathers and their families, can be overlooked. A family history is also important in helping practitioners assess the extent to which they will be able to work in partnership with the father or father figure and whether or not they should be providing services directly to him to alleviate his needs or ensure the protection of the child. These studies found that it was rare for family histories to be prepared in the early stages of contact with the family and six months on from the initial child protection conference. Thoburn *et al.* (1995) found that only 50% of cases had a comprehensive family history on the file, 48% a partial one and 2% none.

Review conferences

The studies noted that review conferences tended to endorse the pattern of case management that had been established. If the original plan had failed to mention how particular interventions with the parents were going to be achieved, the focus quickly moved away from work with the person who had caused the harm on to the difficulties of the children. It is important that reviews are used as an opportunity to challenge these shifts in focus and to ensure that the emphasis remains on achieving good outcomes for children.

Fear of violent men

The fear that professionals have of potentially or actively violent men must be taken seriously. Employers should ensure that there are clear policies in relation to safety and sufficient resources to back up such policies. Providing training to help practitioners deal with their own fear, with aggression and with violent situations is important. O'Hagan and Dillenburger (1995) suggest methods for training social work students in order to assist them in dealing better with situations in which they may feel threatened or fearful. Properly prepared and disciplined role play is important, together with an analysis and understanding of the different ways in which practitioners avoid having to work closely with men, thereby placing extra burdens on women. They point out that in reality social workers are more likely to experience violence from women, because it is with mothers that they have most contact. It is important that workers are offered continuing training to deal with these issues. The probation service, more used to dealing with men, have skills in relation to coping with aggression and with practitioners' fear of aggression and violence that could usefully be passed on to social workers.

Domestic violence

Making an Impact: children and domestic violence training pack (Hester *et al.*, 1998), commissioned by the Department of Health and written by a consortium of practitioners, trainers and researchers from the NSPCC, Barnardo's and the University of Bristol, is designed to ensure that training materials for frontline staff dealing with domestic violence are more readily available than has been the case in the past.

Getting fathers involved

The role of the supervisor and training are important when considering how to get fathers and father figures more involved generally with their children and with the different agencies that are working with their families. Training to help staff work better with fathers needs to be concerned with: self-awareness about personal beliefs, values and prejudices; challenging stereotypes; attitudes to working in a mixed gender team; attitudes to working with fathers; understanding the experiences of fathers and mothers; learning how to value the contribution of fathers; methods of working, for example developing group-work skills and developing a service environment that is friendly to men and women; and being sensitive to the wishes of service users (Ruxton, 1992; European Commission Network on Childcare, 1995).

Summary points

- The research shows that some fathers were engaged or were partners in the process of the child protection enquiries or subsequent work with the family even where allegations were denied or in cases of sexual abuse.

- The fear that professionals feel when working with difficult or dangerous men must be acknowledged and attention given to training and support around these issues.

- There are helpful pointers to the staff training and support required to help agencies working with children in need to engage fathers more routinely in their work (Ruxton, 1992, European Commission Network on Childcare, 1995).

- A training pack is available to assist frontline staff in working with families where there is domestic violence (Hester *et al.*, 1998).

Enhancing children's general quality of life

It is tempting to think that quality of life will be enhanced by separating them from men who are perceived to be the cause of their problems. The studies in *Child Protection: messages from research*, however, show that separation, or legal action, does not **necessarily** lead to better outcomes for children in terms of their overall welfare and development. Better outcomes are achieved when professionals can work in partnership with parents and when attention is given to both the wider welfare needs of children and the needs of their parents and carers. In the majority of cases it will be appropriate to work in partnership with both parents, but in some cases it will be more appropriate to work with the mother only.

- 'The children who derived most benefit from social work intervention were those where social workers (or sometimes other professionals) had succeeded in engaging **both** the children **and** significant parent'; and
- 'A narrow concentration on the child's protection, if it excluded parents' needs, limited the extent to which the child's welfare could be enhanced, since these issues were bound together' (Farmer and Owen, 1995, pp 238 and 287).

Furthermore, it is a mistake to assume that just because a family has serious problems the parents are not committed to the children. Thoburn *et al.* (1995) found that the majority of parents were committed to their children most of the time (p 45) which would indicate that it should be possible to engage fathers. Similarly, Pitcairn *et al.* (1995) found that 90% of mothers and 75% of fathers reported feeling close to their baby (under the age of one) and 63% of both mothers and fathers reported feeling close to their child over the age of one. Overall, 50% of mothers and 35% of fathers spoke glowingly about the child and the vast majority of relationships contained at least some positive elements.

Practitioners should always collect information about the fathers or father figures, and about any men in the household even if they are not playing a fathering role, and should start from the presumption that it will be helpful to engage them in the enquiries and work with the family. But careful assessment will identify those cases where separation is likely to enhance the children's welfare and attempts by social services' staff to work with or engage the father are likely to be counter-productive. In these situations it may be more appropriate to involve professionals from other agencies, such as probation, health or the voluntary sector.

What services are needed?

What sorts of services might be helpful? The studies in *Messages from Research* can do little more than indicate where the gaps are as so few services were directly provided to men. Farmer and Owen's (1995) study showed that at follow-up 70% of children were protected and 68% had their welfare enhanced, but in only 30% of cases were the needs of the main parent or carer met. Thus in only 23% of cases were goals to do with protection, welfare and needs achieved.

Gibbons *et al.* (1995b) found that for children who remained at home, a link with a family centre or voluntary agency was connected with better outcomes for the child in the longer term. This tended to be part of a well-coordinated package of services focusing on particular difficulties. Farmer and Owen identify the interventions that would contribute to the meeting of parents' needs as: the maintenance of links with looked-after children; practical help; work on parent–child relationships; use of mental health services; and mitigation of the ill effects of registration. Cleaver and Freeman (1995) noted that practitioners rarely discussed the range of services that might be available to a family under Section 17, including direct financial help and advice, family therapy, and support and help from other agencies. The research indicates that both mothers and fathers would benefit from help in tackling problems arising from poverty, unemployment and poor housing conditions.

The study by Pitcairn *et al.* (1993) shows a very low incidence of serious injuries to children whose names were placed on the register for physical abuse – mainly bruising and other minor injuries. In their study, what was of more concern was that the research, using Rutter (1967) and Richman *et al.* (1982) child behaviour check lists completed by both parents and professionals, indicated a high level of disturbance in the children. The parents were young and the children had been wanted. The major problem seemed to be lack of control rather than over-disciplining, shouting rather than hitting. The parents acknowledged that they failed to discipline their children when they behaved badly and there was little difference in attitude between the mothers and the fathers. The families were poor, lacking in education and facing other problems (*see* p 46). In view of these facts, it seems clear that the children would benefit more from practical help and support to their parents, and work around parenting skills, than from monitoring of their safety.

Thoburn *et al.* (1995) give an example of work with a family that focused on their individual practical needs as well as on protecting a child:

> A father in an Asian family left home because he had physically abused his child and had mental health problems. He could not manage money. The social worker helped the mother to get her own income support while he was away. When the mother took him back, the social worker helped her keep her own separate income arrangements and arranged for the father to maintain himself financially. The worker offered long-term casework to each family member separately and to the family as a whole – incorporating skilled mental health services for the father with child protection and family support.

The studies reveal that for fathers outside the home almost no help or services are provided. Removing problematic fathers may solve the problem within that particular family but these remain men who have sexually abused a child or who have been violent or aggressive. Many of them will move into new families. Similarly, men who spend time in prison are eventually released. The research studies indicate that some of them return home. It would be helpful if at some point an attempt were made to improve their parenting capacity.

In addition to considering the sorts of services that might be needed for working with these men, there are issues around whether and how the new families they move into are given information about their behaviour towards children in the past. Some local authorities, for example, always let a mother know if they learn that a schedule 1 offender has moved into her home or is having a relationship with her.

In addition to practical assistance and therapeutic work with their relationship problems, the research indicates that the following services would be helpful: anger management; work around domestic violence; parenting skills dealing with both younger children and adolescents; access to counselling and intensive services in relation to alcohol and drug misuse; mental health services; counselling in relation to earlier traumas such as abuse in childhood or the loss of significant adults through rejection or death; and work with perpetrators of sexual abuse.

Making use of other agencies

It is helpful to draw on the expertise of practitioners from other agencies, both for direct work with individual family members and in order to learn from the skills that they have developed. Farmer and Owen (1995) talk about looking to professionals who can work with the disengaged member of the family; if fathers refuse to talk to a police officer, try the health visitor. If the health visitor has no joy, what about a voluntary worker? The range of needs identified in the studies make it clear that other departments within a local authority and other agencies, particularly health and education, but also housing, probation, welfare rights and organisations within the voluntary sector, will be well placed to provide services to meet these needs.

Summary points

- The majority of parents, including fathers, are committed to their children. Practitioners should start from the assumption that it will be helpful to engage fathers in any child protection enquiries and/or work with the family. Careful assessment will identify those cases where attempts to work with or engage the father are likely to be counter-productive.

- Better outcomes are achieved in terms of the overall welfare and development of children if professionals give attention both to the children's wider welfare needs and the needs of their parents and carers.

- Services to meet the needs of fathers should include practical help around housing, employment and money; services to address problems around mental health, alcohol and drug misuse, marital discord, domestic violence, sexual abuse, parenting skills and contact with separated children.

- Removing fathers who have sexually abused or physically injured their children may solve the problem for those particular children, but many of the men move into new families, sometimes after release from prison. Attempts should be made to work with them, which raises the question of who is best placed, or has the responsibility, to carry out this work. If at the time the man is not living with any children is it the responsibility of the social services department? Issues also arise in relation to notifying any new families of the past history of male abusers.

- Other agencies may have skills in working with men that can be be employed. The list of services required to meet the needs of fathers indicates that these are best provided on a multi-agency basis.

Chapter 6

Some examples of services

This final chapter contains some practical examples of services or resources that are available for fathers (*see* Resources, pp 85–8 for contact points). The intention is to give some pointers for practice rather than providing a comprehensive list. Some of the specific projects referred to have been evaluated, some have not. The inclusion of specific projects is for information only and is not an indication that the Department of Health has evaluated them.

Contact between fathers and children

Many children will want continuing contact with fathers or father figures, even in circumstances where those men have harmed them or where there was previous domestic violence. Practitioners should consider each child within the family as they may have different, possibly conflicting, needs in relation to contact. Thoburn *et al.* (1995) give the example of a three-year-old whose father sexually abused his step-daughter, her older half-sister. There was no evidence that he had abused his own daughter but she had no contact with him from the moment that he left the home.

The children's wish for contact may sometimes conflict with their mother's need to be protected from further domestic violence. Research indicates that some fathers use contact to continue their violence against their former partners – by gaining access to her to attack her directly, by harming or threatening to harm the children, or by using the children to pass on threats to her (Hester and Radford, 1996; Hester *et al.*, 1997). Places such as The Meeting Place, run by the **Coram Family**, provide a safe, neutral space for contact. In 1999–2000 similar services were also funded by the Home Office Family Support Grant. Service provision for fathers will be mapped by **Fathers Direct** (*see* list of resources on page 85). Some children who have no wish to see their fathers or father figures may want to have information about them from time to time. In these situations, services are required which will both assist in the promotion of contact or the maintenance of links, while at the same time protecting women and children.

Domestic violence

A variety of methods for changing the behaviour of men who are violent to their partners have been developed over the years. Some of these are specialist schemes, the majority of which have a clear feminist perspective on the issue of male violence, offer support to the women involved at the same time as working with the men, and regard an improved quality of life for the victim as a major criterion of success. Specialist schemes are dependent on funding and/or on receiving referrals from probation services. However, probation are increasingly developing in-house methods of working with violent men which, in some areas can lead to the demise of the specialist scheme.

Some schemes have been evaluated but without measuring the comparative effectiveness of different types of intervention, such as group work as opposed to individual work. An evaluation of two criminal justice-based schemes in Scotland (the **Change Project**, *see* list of resources on page 87; and the **Lothian Domestic Violence Project**) – which deliver structured, cognitive behavioural programmes focusing on the offender and the offending behaviour – found such schemes are more likely than other forms of criminal justice interventions, such as a fine, probation or prison, to eliminate or reduce violent behaviour (Dobash *et al.*, 1996). Men participate in these programmes as a condition of a probation order and attend weekly group sessions for six or seven months. Aspects of the programme that men identified as helping them change were:

- group discussion about attitudes to women
- discussions aimed at teaching them to recognise the 'triggers' associated with their violent acts
- videos depicting familiar scenarios
- homework involving self-monitoring
- learning to take 'time out' to divert them from violent acts.

The West Yorkshire Probation Service has published a booklet which describes group work with men in Wakefield prison serving long or life sentences for rape, murder or sexual abuse of children (West Yorkshire Probation Service; *see* list of resources on page 88).

The Everyman Centre in Plymouth (*see* list of resources on page 87) provides a task-focused, psychosocial counselling programme for men who are violent to women. The majority of men attend the centre on a voluntary basis as a result of self-referral and some men participate as a condition of their probation orders. The centre offers a combination of individual assessment, counselling and group work, over a period of 40–50 weeks. Great importance is attached to the involvement of the partners of the men accepted on to the programme. A reciprocal women's service is offered, providing advice about legal and support services, counselling and psychotherapy, and advice on developing a personal safety strategy if the woman is still living with her partner. Regular contact with partners enables the workers to gauge to what extent the man may be playing down the problem and the seriousness of the risk. It also ensures that men cannot easily lie about their attendance or non-attendance at the centre. The group work focuses on men taking responsibility for their behaviour, helping them to express vulnerability and anger, encouraging an understanding of, and empathy with, the experience of the victims, and looking at alternative ways of behaving. The centre finds that they are very successful in helping men to eliminate their physical violence very quickly, but not necessarily their aggressive, controlling, manipulative behaviour.

The **Domestic Violence Intervention Project** (DVIP *see* list of resources on page 85), like the Everyman Centre, combines working with men with a women's support service. The support service is both for the partners of men on the programme and for women who self-refer. The project was evaluated over a two-year period (Burton *et al.*, 1998) and among the findings from the evaluation were:

- the proactive approach of the women's support service brought women into support services at an earlier stage than would have been the case if the approach had not been made to them
- women did not resent the proactive response, and many of them welcomed it
- over two-thirds of the men referred to the programme did not complete it
- there was a substantial impact on the attitudes and behaviour of the men who did complete the programme.

The researchers evaluating this project expressed concern that the local probation service was shifting funding from this specialist service to running groups for violent men in-house. They pointed out that this could mean a reduced service to men who self-refer and a reduction in linked support for women. They concluded that specialist projects had a number of advantages and that it was important that funding was made available for them.

The **Lawrence Weston Family Centre** in Bristol (*see* list of resources on page 86) works with parents of children in need under the age of five, where there are child protection concerns. In 1989, the centre surveyed 35 of their women clients and found that 30 of them had experienced male violence in the previous 12 months. A group for violent men was set up as a response but there were insufficient referrals to it. The centre decided that working on an individual basis with men could offer a more flexible approach and would be more acceptable to many men. The centre has been working successfully in this way since September 1993. Men are expected, and helped, to accept full responsibility for their behaviour. They are given strategies to avoid and control violence; helped to gain insight into why they behave as they do; the effects of violence on children are explained; and they are helped to become more emotionally articulate. Partners are offered a parallel support service and can contribute to reviews of progress, and in addition couple work is offered at the end of the programme. Men who complete the programme are encouraged to join the centre's fathers' group, and ongoing counselling is available.

Anger management

Evaluations of anger management training indicate that a number of methods are effective in helping to reduce the anger that was leading to the maltreatment of children (Macdonald and Roberts, 1995). Components of these schemes involved:

- helping parents understand their child's behaviour, i.e. it is not a deliberate attempt to annoy them
- teaching them to think of alternative ways of resolving conflicts
- relaxation methods
- a combination of all three of the above.

Macdonald and Roberts point out that anger management training is unlikely to help those whose temper is unpredictable and instantaneous because the methods rely on being able to identify 'triggers'.

Education of men

Working with Men (*see* list of resources on page 88) has received funding to develop a curriculum, materials, strategies and evaluative methods for working with groups of young men (aged 12–18). The aims of the work are to increase awareness of the changing nature of the role of fathers in families; increase their knowledge of the role and responsibilities of being a father; develop young men's skills in aspects of parenthood; and increase confidence in childcare and role negotiation (*Working with Men*, 1997, Vol 2).

The Home Office analysed the effectiveness of parenting courses in young offender institutions. The attitudes of the young men towards enforcing parental discipline showed most susceptibility to change. The courses were successful in suggesting to them a wider range of options than the arbitrary and punitive approaches they expressed to start with (Caddle, 1991).

The **NSPCC** in Barnsley has developed a parenting education programme based on one developed jointly by the NSPCC and Relate in Newcastle. The distinctive feature of the Barnsley scheme is that a group of male volunteers has been recruited and trained to deliver a short parenting education course to 14- and 15-year-old boys in secondary schools. There was no shortage of volunteers for the project. A number of the volunteers are ex-miners, themselves having had to come to terms with major changes in their roles. The volunteers work with groups of eight to ten young men for six sessions over a six-week period. They lead discussions on parenting and relationships. The project was piloted successfully but did not receive funding to continue (Barnsley Parenting Education Project; *see* list of resources on page 85).

Research into the effectiveness of parent training schemes indicates they have good results with a wide range of child behaviour problems, but where there are compounding problems, such as depression, stress, poverty or relationship problems, they are unlikely to provide a sufficient response and longer-term work with the family is also required. Although the research in this area focuses almost exclusively on mothers, the findings have been shown to hold true also for fathers (Macdonald and Roberts, 1995; Patterson *et al.*, 1982; Phares and Compas, 1992).

In the USA, parenting support programmes have begun to develop their curricula to be responsive to different groups of fathers, for example Hispanic fathers or young African-

American fathers (Powell, 1995; Cohen and Ooms, 1994). In New York, the YWCA started a programme for the male partners of the young mothers they were working with. They provided education towards academic qualifications for 16–25-year-old fathers, together with parenting education. In addition, if they wish, fathers receive counselling and have access to the health, fitness and recreational facilities at the centre. Seventy per cent of the fathers who completed the programme actively pursued further education or job training and became more involved parents.

The Government places a high priority on work with fathers. In 1999, *Supporting Families*, a consultation document, was published; it noted that the Ministerial Group on the Family would be looking at ways of encouraging the development of more widespread support for fathers. Work continues to be taken forward in the area of fatherhood.

Child sexual abuse

Currently there is little evidence about the effectiveness of different interventions with adult sexual abusers (Frosh, 1995). Commentators suggest that focused psychotherapeutic work continues alongside more cognitive-behavioural approaches in order to achieve, at least, a better understanding of the nature of abusive behaviour towards children.

The Lucy Faithfull Foundation provides assessments of the non-abusing parent either individually or in addition to assessments of the abuser. They will work with children and their families whether or not the abuser is still in the household. They also provide training and consultancy for other agencies. They apply their knowledge of offenders, and in particular how the offender operated in any specific case, in order to interpret and understand the mother's responses – in relation to the child, the offender and other significant family members. How did he ensure the child did not tell her? If the child did tell, how did he ensure the child was not heard or not believed? If the mother knew about the abuse but did not act, what did he do to ensure that? This information is used to identify the type or types of intervention needed to help the mother protect her child in the future.

In a small number of cases the woman is the abuser. The foundation works with agencies to help identify these cases and provides similar assessments and recommendations for services for non-abusing male partners and fathers of children sexually abused by women or by a man outside the family. The knowledge that most sexual abuse is committed by men, that 50% of convicted female perpetrators are co-offenders with men and that networks of abuse exist, can lead to practitioners making assumptions which in turn feel abusive to those fathers who have not sexually abused their children and knew nothing about the abuse. Such a response undermines those fathers who are trying to support their child through the healing process. The foundation provides an assessment service in cases where there are such suspicions, whereby therapists are able to apply their specialist knowledge of both male and female perpetrators in order to understand and interpret the responses of fathers whose children have been sexually abused. The foundation also provides ongoing support, advice and counselling services for non-abusing fathers either independently or, where the perpetrator is his partner, combined with therapy for the female perpetrator.

The needs of non-abusing men who have a significant relationship with children who have been sexually abused are beginning to be recognised. **Surviving Together** (*see* list of resources on page 87) is a project based in Hackney jointly funded by health, social services and NCH Action for Children. It provides counselling for non-abusing fathers or other males in the family who are important to the child, such as uncles, grandfathers or new partners of the mother. Although the project was initially set up to offer support to women, it has responded to requests to provide support to children and non-abusing men. Referrals are either self-referrals or from professionals such as social workers, health visitors, GPs or the police. The project is for people who live or work in that area and as such the main users are men and women from the black community. It offers both individual

and group counselling. Initially, men have two or three individual sessions and then can then move into a group. The men
set the agenda, the areas of discussion and have a choice of
either a male or female worker. Initially the men are offered
sessions once a week for 12 weeks. Some sessions may be
with couples; sometimes other family members may be
involved (*Community Care*, 1998, 5–11 February).

Fathers' groups and getting fathers involved

There is currently debate and discussion around whether
having male workers in such settings as nurseries and family
centres encourages the greater involvement of fathers both
generally in the care of their children and specifically in
programmes designed to meet their particular needs. There is
some evidence that employing male staff, together with other
strategies does help to involve fathers more (Cohen and Ooms,
1994; Levine, 1993; European Commission Network on
Childcare, 1995; Ghate *et al.*, 2000).

Research carried out in 1991 on the 77 family centres run
by NCH Action for Children (Ruxton, 1992), found that practitioners believed that employing more male workers in family
centres would provide good role models for children and
would also encourage more fathers to make use of the centres
and get more involved in them. The research specifically
focused on male workers in family centres – why there are so
few of them; the characteristics of, and roles performed by,
men who do work in them; how staff and users feel about
their involvement; what may be the advantages and disadvantages of attempting to increase this and how it should be
achieved. The research found that 13% of the full-time and
5% of the part-time workforce was male, as was 16% of the
volunteer group. Women tended to work in the same projects
for much longer than men. In relation to training, a social
work qualification was similarly common among men and
women, but no men had qualifications in nursery and
playgroup work whereas 39% of the qualified female staff
did. A majority of staff (86%) thought that there were not

enough male workers in family centres. The report concluded that there should be positive approaches to recruiting men to family centre work, providing that staff and users were given opportunities to discuss possible areas of concern. The issues that were identified by the research were:

- male workers might be too dominant
- the risk of abuse may increase
- there may be difficulties for children and women who have been sexually abused
- male workers in female-dominated settings need support
- men are not an homogenous group – race, class and sexuality are also important
- team awareness of gender issues is important.

The **Pen Green Centre** in Corby (*see* list of resources on page 87) has had a strategy to involve fathers more in the centre since 1985. Part of that strategy involved recruiting male workers and provides an example of how the above issues can be tackled successfully (European Commission Network on Childcare, 1995). Despite initial anxiety about recruiting male workers – would they take over? How would it affect abused women and children or women who enjoyed the male-free environment? – the centre has now concluded that children are entitled to access to male workers; that children need the example of positive male role models; and that staff groups also benefit from being mixed. Having male workers is also important for effective work with both fathers and mothers. The centre's strategy has resulted in more fathers bringing and collecting their children and taking part in the week-long settling in period required by the nursery and an increased involvement by fathers in groups at the centre. In relation to concerns about possible abuse of children by male staff, the centre emphasises the importance of better training for staff, parents and children on assertiveness and improper touching, and of an open and non-hierarchical approach to working.

The initial action plan at Pen Green had as its objectives: to raise awareness within parents' groups of ways in which women keep men out of places such as family centres and to explore the positive reasons why women want a place of their own; to develop staff training on gender issues and to get staff to reflect on their own feelings about men in the nursery; and to develop direct work with fathers.

The practical action taken included making the centre more 'men friendly', for example by displaying photos of fathers with their children; videoing how staff greeted mothers and fathers when they brought their children to the centre; visiting fathers at home and discussing their involvement in the home and how they would like to use Pen Green; formally writing to fathers and inviting them to attend meetings; positive action in advertising specifically for male workers.

Additional objectives developed since 1990 include: to examine why fathers find it difficult to commit to groups; to look at gender issues in relation to the leadership of groups; to experiment with male staff making direct contact with fathers through home visits and group work focused on fathers' parenting issues; to study how fathers and male workers play with children in the centre; to understand better how fathers see their role.

Meeting these objectives involved more staff training; groups being co-led by men and women; and broadening the range of groups and activities in the centre available to men. There is a well-established men's group for fathers of children at the centre, to enable the fathers (mainly working-class men) to explore a range of personal issues.

The strategy to involve fathers has been a continuous and interactive process, essential elements of which have been: staff training; research (for example, into staff attitudes and belief systems, and into what fathers themselves wanted from the centre); and constant evaluation of the services offered.

Evaluations of setting up fathers' groups or of getting men more involved in a project, family centre or nursery both in this country and in the USA give some consistent messages.

- Getting fathers to come to groups is difficult, time-consuming and can be costly – both for self-referrals and referrals from other agencies.

- There is a high drop-out rate from some groups, but workers should not necessarily lose heart because of this.
- Having a small, core group of committed fathers is important.
- Fathers may need to be followed up persistently – failure to respond to letters and phone calls may not indicate lack of motivation; more often it indicates scepticism that the 'helping agencies' have anything to offer.
- Having male staff is helpful, and using them to make direct contact with fathers, often via home visits, can help engage fathers.
- Making fathers feel welcome – the way staff behave to them; pictures on the walls of fathers, grandfathers, etc.; ensuring meetings are arranged at times when fathers can attend.
- Staff training on gender issues.
- Keeping mothers fully informed about any work in relation to fathers and working with mothers on issues that might help them.
- Recognising that fathers are not a homogenous group – there are differences of age, class, race, sexuality.

The Lawrence Weston Family Centre in Bristol encourages agencies to identify the needs of fathers as well as mothers at referral stage. It tries to ensure that fathers are involved in all introductory visits so that during this initial phase they are offered the same range of services as mothers. Workers spend time with fathers on their own to enable them to develop their trust in the workers before expecting them to attend a group.

NEWPIN (*see* list of resources on page 87) is a national voluntary organisation with a network of 16 day centres which aim to break down the cyclical effects of destructive family behaviour by supporting adults and pre-school children who have suffered emotional and physical abuse. Very few fathers used NEWPIN's mainstream services prior to the start of its fathers' groups in 1997. Beginning in September 1997, NEWPIN's first fathers' support group ran for 30 weekly sessions. The 'graduates' of that group went on to complete a six-week course in befriending skills to enable them to become mentors for the fathers joining the next group which started at the end of the following year. The goals of the group are:

- to enhance fathers' understanding of the developmental and emotional needs of children and to promote the acquisition of specific skills, knowledge and attitudes that foster competent parenting
- to do this in a reflective and supportive framework that addresses the personal and social issues which shape parenting and family relationships.

Any man with an important role in caring for a child or children can apply to join – whether they are resident or non-resident, lone parents or part of a couple. The group runs for 28 weekly sessions of two and a half hours. The group meets periodically at weekends with the children and, where appropriate adult partners, for lunch, play activities and informal outings.

As with many such groups getting the referrals was a very slow and time-consuming business. Most statutory, voluntary and community organisations receiving publicity about the project expressed enthusiasm but said they had little active involvement with fathers. Some agencies indicated that fathers were unwilling to make use of services, but NEWPIN found that this image of reluctant fathers was misleading. Many fathers were wary of services for families and did not expect them to be supportive, but became motivated and committed to the group once they had met and built up trust in a particular worker.

Successful referrals were often the result of active and sustained encouragement by the referring agency, followed up proactively by NEWPIN. However, half the referrals dropped out before they were interviewed. The interview itself, between the coordinator and the father, was a crucial forum for establishing trust and maintaining the fathers' interest in the group. Nearly two-thirds of those interviewed signed up for the group. Most of those joining had some prior experience of counselling or therapy, usually in a group setting.

In general, the men lacked practical experience and confidence in caring for children. Their main goals were: sharing experiences and feeling less alone; gaining confidence as a parent; exploring the impact of their upbringing on their parenting; learning to look after themselves and not having unrealistic expectations of themselves as a father; understanding their children better; learning how to control angry feelings; and getting practical advice on how to handle difficult situations. They also shared a general feeling that they did not want to repeat the poor parenting (particularly by their fathers) that they had experienced.

The group was facilitated by two project workers, one male and one female. NEWPIN's intention here was to provide a model of how a man and a woman could negotiate and cooperate effectively and to facilitate the process of discussing gender within the group, and this was achieved.

It is clear from information gathered through the initial and end-of-group interviews that the men valued it highly and nearly all of them said they had made substantial changes in their relationship with their children. They felt less bound up in feelings of anger and shame about the past, more confident and were more aware of their children's needs.

Beginning in early 1999, NEWPIN set up shorter (eight-week), less intensive fathers' support groups which consist of free-standing modules and drop-in groups as well as a gateway to the longer programme for those who choose to join it. Such a structure could be used for specific subgroups of fathers – black and ethnic minority fathers; fathers in prison or on probation; young fathers or non-resident fathers. NEWPIN plan to employ a black male worker to develop short programmes for black fathers in South East London.

A support group in Swindon (**KOALAS**) for parents of children with special needs received a project grant from the Department of Health to set up and evaluate a group for fathers (*see* list of resources on page 86). The group had identified that although their philosophy was to provide support to the whole family, they were in fact only in contact with mothers. The fathers' group met once a week in the evenings and once a month on a Saturday morning when the fathers were encouraged to bring their children so they could watch the children play and get involved in activities with them together with staff. The evaluation found that although attendance at meetings varied and was often low, there was a small, core group of committed fathers who kept attending and who may be able to begin to offer support to other fathers. Changing the days of the evening meetings allowed more fathers to attend. They welcomed the opportunity to meet other fathers and to talk to professionals about a range of issues, including employment and dealing with health professionals, as well as their feelings about their children. Friendships were formed enabling whole families to get together with others who had children with special needs.

Projects set up in the USA designed to help young unmarried fathers gain employment, apart from experiencing the common difficulties of attracting young fathers on to the schemes, found that those who did attend responded to the focus on fatherhood. Forty per cent (of 228 fathers) said they enrolled to improve their relationships with their children and 50% said they wanted to improve their parenting skills (Watson, 1992).

In the early 1990s, the Headstart programme in the USA funded projects specifically to get fathers and significant other males in families to be more involved in the programmes.

Elements of successful schemes included:

- appointing male workers to contact fathers directly
- programmes around parenting and other issues specifically designed for different cultural groups
- group discussions providing information on building self-esteem; child development; legal rights; adult education; and advice about employment and health, including mental health and substance misuse
- making sure mothers were fully informed about the programmes and that they supported the increased involvement of men

(Cohen and Ooms, 1994; Levine, 1993).

Fathers' Direct

In its proposals for public policy in relation to fathers, the Institute for Public Policy Research (Burgess and Ruxton, 1996) recommended the setting up of a Fathers' Resource Centre, similar to the Families and Work Institute in the USA (*see* list of resources on page 85). The centre would act as a focal point for the collection, analysis and distribution of information for and about the needs of fathers with information, among other things, about national and local organisations offering advice and support. In 1999, Fathers Direct was launched. This organisation provides information direct to fathers and to those working with them, as well as working on policy development and, together with other organisations, piloting initiatives aimed to improve fathers' access to services (*see* pp 85–8). It has been funded by the Home Office Family Support Grant to raise the awareness of the role of the fathers and change the public perception of fatherhood. It has developed a web site (www.fathersdirect.org) for fathers and is working with Parentline Plus on making its helpline for parents attractive and relevant to fathers. It has worked with Bounty to produce a pack for new fathers: *Bounty Guide to Fatherhood*. Fathers Direct is working with others to map services available to fathers (*see* pp 85–8).

The Home Office is providing approximately £7 million over a three year period through the Family Support Grant to voluntary organisations working with families. In 1999, it concentrated on work with boys, young men and fathers. Fathers Direct was funded, as were a number of other organisations which support fathers.

Conclusions

There is by now a considerable body of information on the lives of children in need. Yet reading through the books in the Department of Health Child Protection series and other relevant research, one struggles to find much on the men in children's lives. One reason, noted at the outset, is the simple one that none of the research focuses on fathers specifically; professionals tend to collect relatively little about them when they are gathering information about families, but it remains a serious omission that needs to be rectified.

Figure 1 on page 33 provides a reasonable starting point. We need to ask: Who are the father figures in the child's life? Are they resident or absent? Are they a risk to the child or a potential protective agent? Are they interested in the child or remote? Knowing who the father is and where he lives – building up a reasonable social history explaining his relationship with the child and other family members – provides important information when working with children and their families.

The studies show that the inevitable consequence of failure to engage with men implicated in the maltreatment of their children, whether they lived inside or outside the home, was their under-involvement in the decision-making process. 'In terms of the accurate diagnosis of risk this could be considerable disadvantage. An additional problem is that when moves are made towards more contractual working, we need to consider with whom the agreement needs to be made' (Farmer and Owen, 1995, p 109). In short, a failure to involve a man implicated in maltreatment means that the needs of his child and family are seldom adequately met. Farmer and Owen note that male abusers who presented risks to children or partners tended to opt out of social work involvement and as a result their problems were not directly addressed (p 320). Other commentators have noted the variety of ways in which practitioners avoid men (O'Hagan and Dillenburger, 1995).

However they behave, fathers, whether they be absent or present, are a significant part of the lives of most children in need and the research studies suggest that it is difficult to achieve optimal outcomes without including the man as at least the subject – if not an active participant – of professional deliberation.

Engaging with fathers is not beyond the powers of individual practitioners. The key is to identify the source of children's needs and understand the fathers' roles in their lives – rather than categorising them only as either perpetrator or non-perpetrator – and to consider how to ensure that a father's involvement promotes the child's best interests. Fathers are not a homogenous group; there are differences arising from ethnicity, culture, class, age and sexuality. In addition, as these studies have shown, there are fathers and father figures in the home and out of the home, in contact or not with their children, who have a range of different needs, who may be abusive or neglectful to their partners or children, or who may sexually abuse their own children or the children of others, or who may be distant and unsupportive, or who may be warm and supportive parents. In fact, for many groups of children in need, especially those requiring practical support, housing or advice with parenting, fathers seek the same help as mothers and often their participation in any plan is vital to its success.

Whether the deliberation is specific – about a particular case – or general – about a group of cases coming to notice in a local authority – thinking will be made easier by concentrating on outcomes in the context of children's needs. What is it we are trying to achieve for this child or group of children? Where do we want to get to in six weeks, six months or a year's time? What services are we going to put into place to achieve these outcomes? And how will family members – including fathers – be involved to get the best out of these services?

By concentrating on outcomes, the purpose of different strategies, say engaging men in family centres or nurseries, psychological programmes to improve anger management or excluding men from the family home, becomes manifest. Men contribute to (and alleviate) children's needs in different ways, a finding that should be built into the organisation and delivery of children's services.

This said, tensions are likely to persist until there is an articulate and broadly supported view of men's role in modern family life. Being a father in 2000 is different from being a father in 1960. Although many fathers continue to have the role of breadwinner, the traditional model of the breadwinning father and stay-at-home, caring mother is not supported by half the population. There is debate and discussion among professionals working with children and among policy makers about the need to recognise the caring responsibilities of fathers and their role in children's development. Privately within families there is negotiation and/or disagreement about who should be doing what, when and why. For families in contact with social services there may be the additional tensions of poverty, poor housing, racism, physical and mental health problems, and lack of access to good childcare and to leisure facilities. These additional pressures need to be taken account of when designing services for fathers and considering ways of engaging them in their children's lives.

The implications of these conclusions for practice and for policy can be summarised as follows.

Summary of conclusions – practice issues

- Although there is a lot of interest generally in fathers and their role in families and influence on children's development, in the past little was done by any of the childcare agencies systematically to engage father and father figures. Interest has been growing and services are being developed. It is of note that in 1999 many applicants to the Family Support Grant were asking for resources to start local work on how to engage fathers.

- The evidence from studies looking at the child protection system shows that professionals focus on mothers. Partly this is because professionals do not attempt to find out about or engage with fathers, partly it is because fathers distance themselves. This is not a problem specific to social services but applies to other agencies working with children and families as well.

- There should be a presumption that working with and engaging the father will benefit the child, but careful assessment in individual cases will identify the circumstances where attempts to engage the father by social work staff would be counter-productive. Making use of the skills and resources of other agencies may well be appropriate in these cases.

- In order to work with fathers professionals need to find out more about them – their role in the family, relationship (legal and otherwise) to the children and, if they are non-resident, the level and nature of their continuing involvement in their children's lives, risk and protective factors in their relationship with their children and details of their own needs.

- Training and support is required on how better to engage fathers in the care of their children and in working with childcare agencies, and also on how to work with violent or aggressive men and to cope with the fear they provoke. This should include inter-agency and post-qualifying training. Practitioners need to be given the opportunity to make use of, or learn from, the skills of professionals in other agencies.

- Services to respond to the needs of fathers should be provided.

Summary of conclusions – policy

- Research in the area of children in need should in future treat parents as separate entities, identifying who was interviewed and to whom a particular observation refers. It should also distinguish between the perpetrating and the potentially non-abusing parent and between fathers and father figures. It is important to collect information from fathers as well as from mothers, children and professionals. It would also be helpful to collect information from and about fathers from different minority ethnic groups.

- Future policy developments, for example those around early preventive services, should recognise the positive role that fathers can play in child development and should also recognise the lack of services which are father friendly or which encourage them to engage with the agencies providing services to their children.

- Agencies should be given support in working with, or attempting to work with, father or father figures who have been violent to, or have sexually abused, children but who are not living in the family at that time and who have not been convicted of an offence.

Studies in the Department of Health Child Protection Research Programme

Farmer E and Owen M (1995) *Child Protection Practice: private risks and public remedies.* HMSO, London.

Research carried out in two local authorities. A quantitative survey of case conference decision making, planning and process. 120 initial case conferences were attended during 1989 and 1990. 44 children placed on the register (60% of those registered) were followed up. Parents, key workers and older children were interviewed twice, once soon after the conference and again 20 months later. All 44 mothers were interviewed and one third (14) of the fathers or father figures. Ten further cases were selected from a third local authority to provide a small sample of children from a minority ethnic background.

Thoburn J, Lewis A and Shemmings D (1995) *Paternalism or Partnership? Family involvement in the child protection process.* HMSO, London.

The study comprised 220 cases in seven local authorities identified after the initial child protection conference. In 68% of these cases the child was registered. Case records were examined six months after the conference and questionnaires completed by the main carer and the social worker. A small sample of 33 families was followed up. 58% of children in this sample were registered. The researchers attended the case conferences, interviewed the families and the workers. 28 mothers or stepmothers were interviewed and 15 fathers or stepfathers. In the small and large samples 15% (five and 33 children) of the children were from minority ethnic groups.

Cleaver H and Freeman P (1995) *Parental Perspectives in Cases of Suspected Child Abuse*. HMSO, London.

This is an analysis of all incidents of suspected child abuse in one area in one year – 583 cases. In 29% of cases the child's name was placed on the register. The referrals came from a range of different agencies, whose files were examined. 30 families with 61 children thought to be at risk, and the professionals, were interviewed over a two-year period from the concerns first emerging. 23% (seven) of the families in the small sample were from minority ethnic groups.

Gibbons J, Conroy S and Bell C (1995a) *Operating the Child Protection System: a study of child protection practices in English local authorities*. HMSO, London.

This was a study of 1888 referrals raising child protection concerns in eight local authority social services departments.

Gibbons J, Gallagher B, Bell C and Gordon D (1995b) *Development After Physical Abuse in Early Childhood*. HMSO, London.

A follow-up study of all children under five whose names were placed on the Child Protection Register in 1981 in two areas. There were 170 children in the sample. There was also a matched comparison group. The circumstances of the abuse and registration were obtained from agency records as was the situation of the children five years on from registration. The research was conducted ten years after registration and the situation of the children was elicited from interviews with main carers, older children, teachers and social workers, questionnaires and testing. Of the index children 11% were mixed parentage, 5% were black and 2% were Asian. The comparable figures for the comparison group were 5%, 3% and 2%.

ESRC funded study:

Sharland E, Seal H, Croucher M, Aldgate J and Jones D (1995) *Professional Intervention in Child Sexual Abuse.* HMSO, London.

This study looked at all referrals for sexual abuse concerns to the police and the social services department in one area over a nine-month period. The survey group comprised 220 children from 147 families and from that group 34 families with 41 children were interviewed. Parents, children and professionals were interviewed once in the early weeks of the investigation and once again 12 months on. Among the criteria for selecting families for interview were that the investigation had proceeded to at least one professional interview with the child and that the children were suspected or confirmed to have been abused or at risk, but not to have perpetrated abuse. The study did not distinguish between mothers and fathers or father figures when reporting on the interview findings.

Pitcairn T, Waterhouse L, McGhee J, Secker J and Sullivan C (1993) Evaluating parenting in child physical abuse. In: L Waterhouse (ed) *Child Abuse and Child Abusers*, pp 73–92. Jessica Kingsley, London.

This ESRC funded study looked at 43 cases of physical abuse in three regional departments of social work in Scotland. In all cases the index child was under 12 and there was no psychotic disorder in the parents. All the children were the subject of child protection conferences, but not all were registered. Parents were interviewed shortly after the conference and again four months later. Social workers were also interviewed. Parents and professionals completed Rutter and Richman check lists on the children. Mothers were the main informants – 40 mothers were interviewed and 12 fathers.

Smith M, Bee P, Heverin A and Nobes G (1993) *Parental Control Within the Family: the nature and extent of parental violence to children.* Thomas Coram Research Unit, London.

The study focused on 403 families drawn at random from the total population in two geographical areas. Each family selected had a child in one of four age groups – one, four, seven or 11 years. The researchers interviewed 403 mothers, 99 fathers and 215 children. The interviews covered three main areas: the nature and extent of punishment of children, factors which may be associated with high levels of physical punishment and the parent/child relationship and child behaviour.

Resources

Barnsley Parenting Education Project
This project was piloted by:
NSPCC
9 Churchfield Court
Barnsley S70 2JT
Tel: 01226 779494

Domestic Violence Intervention Project (DVIP)
PO Box 2838
London W6 9ZE
Tel: 020 8563 7983

Families and Work Institute
330 Seventh Avenue
New York City
NY 10001
USA
Tel: (212) 465 2044
Fax: (212) 465 8637

Fathers Direct
Tamarisk House
37 The Televillage
Crickhowell NP8 1BP
Tel: 01873 810515
Fax: 01873 810633
email: mail@fathersdirect.org
Contact: Duncan Fisher

Fathers Plus
Children North East
1A Claremont Street
Newcastle upon Tyne NE2 4AH
Tel: 0191 221 0456
Contact: Alan Richardson
> This project was established in 1997 to develop a variety of
> approaches to supporting and empowering fathers including
> establishing a network of people with an interest and/or
> experience of working with fathers. The project has published
> a helpful guide to current projects: *An Audit of Work With
> Fathers Throughout the North East of England: 1998*
> (Richardson, 1998).

KOALAS Swindon Opportunity Group
Rec Room
Victoria Hospital
Okus Road
Old Town
Swindon
Wiltshire SN1 4HZ
Tel: 01793 615351
(Support group for children with special needs)

Lawrence Weston Family Centre
Home Farm
King's Watson Lane
Bristol BS11 0JE
Tel: 0117 982 4578

**Levine J and Pitt E (1996) *New Expectations: community
strategies for responsible fatherhood*. Families and
Work Institute, New York.**
> Contains a review of the research on fathers, looks at the
> critical role of women; profiles effective programmes and
> strategies; and contains a directory of programmes and an
> annotated guide to the most useful books and articles on the role
> of fathers.

Lothian Domestic Violence Project
Domestic Violence Probation Project (DVPP)
Central Criminal Justice Services
1 Parliament Square
Edinburgh EH1 1RF
Tel: 0131 469 3408
Contacts: Moira Andrew and Rory McCrae

National NEWPIN
Sutherland House
35 Sutherland Square
London SE17 3EE
Tel: 020 7703 6376
Contact re Fathers Group: David Bartlett

Parentline Plus
Tel: 0808 800 2222

Pen Green Centre
Pen Green Lane
Corby
Northamptonshire NN17 1BJ
Contact: Trevor Chandler

Programmes on Men's Violence Towards Women
The Change Project
4–6 South Lumley Street
Grangemouth
Stirling FK3 8BT

Surviving Together
Project Director: Cynthia Kelchure-Cole
Tel: 020 7301 3154/6
See Community Care 1998, 5–11 February

The Everyman Centre
6 Victoria Place
Millbay Road
Plymouth PL1 3LP
Tel: 01752 222922
Contact: Calvin Bell

The Lucy Faithfull Foundation
Windmill House
Weatheroak Hill
Alvechurch
Birmingham B48 7EA
Tel: 01564 822446

The Meeting Place
Coram Family
49 Mecklenburgh Square
London WC1N 2QA
Tel: 020 7520 0300

West Yorkshire Probation Service
Why Do Men Commit Most Crime? Focusing on masculinity in a prison group
Available from: The Library WYPS, CLH Hill House, Sandy Walk, Wakefield, West Yorkshire WF1 2JD. Tel: 01924 364141.

Working with Men
320 Commercial Way
London SE15 1QN
Editors: Trefor Lloyd and Tristan Wood
Published four times a year and available by subscription only. Focuses on practice and practice issues for professionals working with men around issues of masculinity, sexism, violence and sexual abuse. It contains features on practice and research. *WWM* also sell publications and produce resources for working with men and boys.

References

Batchelor J, Dimock B and Smith D (1994) *Understanding Step-families: what can be learned from callers to the step-family counselling service?* Step-Family Publications, National Step-family Association, London.

British Household Panel Survey (BHPS) (1990–92). BHPS, Colchester.

Bradshaw J, Stimson C, Williams J and Skinner C (1997) *Non-resident Fathers in Britain*. Paper presented to ERSC Pro- gramme on Population and Household Change Seminar, 13th March.

Brandon M and Lewis A (1996) Significant harm and children's experiences of domestic violence. *Child and Family Social Work*. 1: 33–42.

Brown A (1982) Fathers in the labour ward: medical and lay accounts. In: L McKee and M O'Brien (eds) *The Father Figure*. Tavistock, London.

Burgess A (1997) *Fatherhood Reclaimed: the making of the modern father*. Vermilion, London.

Burgess A and Ruxton S (1996) *Men and Their Children: proposals for public policy*. Institute for Public Policy Research, London.

Burghes L, Clarke L and Cronin N (1997) *Fathers and Fatherhood in Britain*. Family Policy Studies Centre, London.

Burton S, Regan L and Kelly L (1998) *Supporting Women and Challenging Men: lessons from the domestic violence intervention project*. Policy Press, Bristol.

Caddle D (1991) *Parenthood Training for Young Offenders: an evaluation of courses in young offender institutions*. Home Office Research and Planning Unit, Paper 63. HMSO, London.

Children Act 1989. HMSO, London.

Clarke L (1997) Unpublished analysis of 1991 National Child Development Study Data.

Cleaver H and Freeman P (1995) *Parental Perspectives in Cases of Suspected Child Abuse.* HMSO, London.

Cohen E and Ooms T (1994) *Looking Ahead: the promise of Head Start as a comprehensive family support programme.* A Background Briefing Report. Family Impact Seminar, Washington DC.

Court Service (2000) *Court Service Statistics.*

Department of Health (1995a) *Child Protection: messages from research.* HMSO, London.

Department of Health, Social Services Inspectorate (1995b) *The Challenge of Partnership in Child Protection: practice guide.* HMSO, London.

Department of Health (2000a) *Children Looked After by Local Authorities. Year Ending 21 March 1999. England.* Government Statistical Services, London.

Department of Health (2000b) *The Children Act Report 1995–99.* The Stationery Office, London.

Department of Health (1999) *Children and Young People on Child Protection Registers. Year Ending 31 March 1999. England.* Government Statistical Service, London.

Department of Health, Home Office, Department for Education and Employment (1999) *Working Together to Safeguard Children: a guide to inter-agency working to safeguard and promote the welfare of children.* The Stationery Office, London.

Department of Health, Department for Education and Employment, Home Office (2000) *Framework for the Assessment of Children in Need and their Families.* The Stationery Office, London.

Department of Health and Cleaver H (2000) *Assessment Recording Forms.* The Stationery Office, London.

Dobash R, Dobash R, Cavanagh K and Lewis R (1996) *Research Evaluation of Programmes for Violent Men.* The Stationery Office, Edinburgh.

European Commission Network on Childcare (1995) *Fathers, Nurseries and Childcare.* Thomas Coram Research Unit, London.

Family Rights Group (1991) *The Children Act 1989: working in partnership with families.* FRG, London.

Farmer E and Owen M (1995) *Child Protection Practice: private risks and public remedies.* HMSO, London.

Farmer E and Owen M (1998) Gender and the child protection process. *British Journal of Social Work.* **28**: 545–64.

Ferri E and Smith K (1996) *Parenting in the 1990s.* Family and Parenthood Series. Family Policy Studies Centre, London.

Frosh S (1995) Characteristics of sexual abusers. In: K Wilson and A James (eds) *The Child Protection Handbook.* Baillière Tindall, London.

Gershuny J (1996) Unpublished data. ESRC Research Centre on Micro-Social Change, University of Essex.

Ghate D, Shaw C and Hazel N (2000) *Fathers and Family Centres: engaging fathers in preventive services.* Policy Research Bureau, London.

Gibbons J, Conroy S and Bell C (1995a) *Operating the Child Protection System: a study of child protection practices in English local authorities.* HMSO, London.

Gibbons J, Gallagher B, Bell C and Gordon D (1995b) *Development After Physical Abuse in Early Childhood.* HMSO, London.

Hester M and Radford L (1996) *Domestic Violence and Child Contact Arrangements in England and Denmark.* Policy Press, Bristol.

Hester M, Pearson C and Harwin N (1998) *Making an Impact: children and domestic violence. A reader.* Barnados, Ilford.

Hester M, Pearson C and Radford L (1997) *Domestic Violence: a national survey of court welfare and voluntary sector mediation practice.* Policy Press, Bristol.

Jackson B (1984) *Fatherhood.* Allen and Unwin, London.

Kempson E (1996) *Life On a Low Income.* Joseph Rowntree Foundation, York.

Lamb M (ed) (1997) *The Role of the Father in Child Development* (3e). Wiley, Chichester.

Levine J (1993) Involving fathers in Head Start: a framework for public policy and program development in families in society. *The Journal of Contemporary Human Services.* **January**: 4–18.

Lewis C and O'Brien M (eds) (1987) *Reassessing Fatherhood.* Sage, London.

Lord Chancellor's Department (1998) *Court Procedures for the Determination of Paternity and The Law on Parental Responsibility for Unmarried Fathers.* Consultation document.

Macdonald G and Roberts H (1995) *What Works in the Early Years?* Barnados, Ilford.

Marsh P (1987) Social work and fathers: an exclusive practice? In: C Lewis and MJ O'Brien (eds) *Reassessing Fatherhood.* Sage, London.

Marsh P and Crow G (1998) *Family Group Conferences in Child Welfare*. Blackwell Science, Oxford.

Mullender A and Morley R (eds) (1994) *Children Living with Domestic Violence*. Whiting and Birch, London.

Nobes G and Smith M (1997) Physical punishment of children in two-parent families. *Clinical Child Psychology and Psychiatry*. **2**: 271–81.

Nobes G and Smith M (2000) The relative extent of physical punishment and abuse by mothers and fathers. *Trauma, Violence and Abuse*. **1**(1).

Office of National Statistics (1997) *Social Focus on Families*. The Stationery Office, London.

Office for National Statistics (2000) *1998 Birth Statistics Series FMI No. 27*. Government Statistical Service, London.

O'Hagan K and Dillenburger K (1995) *The Abuse of Women within Childcare Work*. The Open University, Milton Keynes.

Patterson G, Chamberlain P and Reid J (1982) A comparative evaluation of a parent training programme. *Behaviour Therapy*. **13**: 638–50

Phares V (1996) *Fathers and Developmental Psychopathology*. Wiley, Chichester.

Phares V (1997) Psychological adjustment, maladjustment and father–child relationships. In: M Lamb (ed) *The Role of the Father in Child Development* (3e). Wiley, Chichester.

Phares V and Compas B (1992) The role of fathers in child and adolescent psychopathology: make room for daddy. *Psychological Bulletin*. **3**: 387–412.

Pitcairn T, Waterhouse L, McGhee J, Secker J and Sullivan C (1993) Evaluating parenting in child physical abuse. In: L Waterhouse (ed) *Child Abuse and Child Abusers*, pp 73–92. Jessica Kingsley, London.

Pleck J (1982) *Husbands' and Wives' Paid Work, Family Work and Adjustment*. Wellesley College Centre for Research on Women, Wellesley.

Pleck J (1983) Husbands' paid work and family roles: current research issues. In: H Lopata and J Pleck (eds) *Research in the Interweave of Social Roles, vol 3, Families and Jobs*. JAI, Greenwich, CT, pp 231–333.

Powell D (1995) Involving Latino fathers in parent education and support programmes. In: R Zambrano (ed) *Understanding Latino Families: scholarship, policy and practice*. Sage, Sacramento, CA.

Quinn R and Staines G (1979) *The 1997 Quality of Employment Survey*. Survey Research Centre, Ann Arbor, MI.

Richman N, Stevenson J and Graham PJ (1982) *Preschool to School: a behavioural study*. Academic Press, London.

Rutter M (1967) A children's behaviour questionnaire for completion by teachers: preliminary findings. *Journal of Child Psychology and Psychiatry*. **8**: 1–11.

Ruxton S (1992) *What's He Doing at the Family Centre?* National Children's Home, London.

Sharland E, Seal H, Croucher M, Aldgate J and Jones D (1995) *Professional Intervention in Child Sexual Abuse*. HMSO, London.

Shulman S and Seiffge-Krenke I (1996) *Fathers and Adolescents: developmental and clinical perspectives*. Routledge, London.

Skuse D, Bentovim A, Hodges J, Stevenson J *et al.* (1998) Risk factors for development of sexually abusive behaviour in sexually victimised adolescent boys: cross-sectional study. *BMJ*. **317**: 175–9.

Sternberg K (1997) Fathers: the missing parents in research on family violence. In: M Lamb (ed) *The Role of the Father in Child Development* (3e). Wiley, Chichester.

Thoburn J, Lewis A and Shemmings D (1995) *Paternalism or Partnership? Family involvement in the child protection process*. HMSO, London.

Thoburn J, Brandon M, Lewis A and Way A (2000) *Safeguarding Children within the Children Act 1989*. The Stationery Office, London. In press.

Watson BH (1992) *Young Unwed Fathers Pilot Project. Initial Implementation Report*. Public/Private Ventures, Philadelphia, PA.

Index